INTERMITTENT FASTING

FOR WOMEN BIBLE

8 BOOKS IN 1

Beginner's Collection For Rapid
Weight Loss, Fat Burning And A
Healthy Lifestyle For Women

By

Beatrice Anahata

and

Heather Trill

damages, or monetary loss due to the information herein, either directly or indirectly.

Respective authors own all copyrights not held by the publisher.

The information herein is offered for informational purposes solely, and is universal as so. The presentation of the information is without contract or any type of guarantee assurance.

The trademarks that are used are without any consent, and the publication of the trademark is without permission or backing by the trademark owner. All trademarks and brands within this book are for clarifying purposes only and are the owned by the owners themselves, not affiliated with this document.

Table of Contents

Book 1: Intermittent Fasting for Women

A Simple 14-Day Beginner's Guide to Fast Weight Loss, Fat Burn, and A Healthy Longer Life.

By

Beatrice Anahata

Introduction

What Is Intermittent Fasting?

Intermittent fasting can be described as alternating intervals of feeding periods and not eating (fasting) period. It simply means you alternate a feeding window and a fasting window. The length of time for each window will vary heavily depending on the protocol of fasting you adopt.

Your body is structured for a smooth transition between fasted and fed states. When in the fed state the level of insulin is elevated thereby signaling the body to store all excess calories in fat cells. The burning of fat is also halted, and the body burns the glucose from your previous meal instead. On the other hand, when your body is in the fasted state insulin levels drop, and hormones that oppose insulin (growth and glucagon hormones) are elevated. This forces the body to burn fat stored in the fat cells to produce energy. This simply means burning fat can only happen when the body is in the fasted state and store more fat when in the fed state.

The moment you begin eating your body enters into the fed state, for the next 3-5 hours the works on the food you consume. The level of insulin in your body rises significantly thereby shutting off fat burning and storing the excess calories. After the mentioned hours the body will enter the post-absorptive state. In the absorptive state, the body is still circulating the components from the last meal you ate. The postabsorptive state last for 8-12 hours after the last meal taken. It takes 12 hours for your body to go into the fasted state fully.

The idea behind intermittent fasting is eating ad libitum when the feeding window opens and when the fasting window starts you avoid drinking or eating stuff with caloric value, but tea or coffee sweetened with erythritol or stevia are allowed. What this means is eating to satiety without compromising your daily macronutrients levels.

You might be new to the concept of intermittent fasting, but you have practiced a form of fasting before. The difference is that in most cases you fast haphazardly i.e. you do not follow a structured fasting timetable, and for this reason, you end up gaining no benefit.

For example, sleeping can be described as a fasting window. When you are sleeping you practice a fairly rigid period of fasting which can last for 6-8 hours per night before you take your breakfast. This is the reason your first meal for the day is called breakfast (breaking your overnight fast).

By nature, intermittent fasting is intermittent and is no way remotely similar to anorexia. This is because IF is done for controlled periods which are brief whereas anorexia an extreme caloric restriction sustained with a goal to lose fat extremely fast. One of the best examples of intermittent fasting is Ramadan; practiced for 4 weeks by Muslims.

Intermittent Fasting for Women

For women who are interested in weight loss, intermittent fasting may seem like a great choice, but many people want to know, should women fast? Is intermittent fasting effective for women? There have been a few critical studies about intermittent fasting which can help to shed some light on this interesting new dietary trend.

Intermittent fasting is also known as alternate-day fasting, although there are certainly some variations on this diet. The American Journal of Clinical Nutrition performed a study recently that enrolled 16 obese men and women in a 10-week program. On the fasting days, participants consumed food to 25% of their estimated energy needs. The rest of the time, they received dietary counseling but were not given a specific guideline to follow during this time.

As expected, the participants lost weight due to this study, but what researchers found interesting were some specific changes. The subjects were all still obese after just 10 weeks, but they had shown improvement in cholesterol, LDL-cholesterol, triglycerides, and systolic blood pressure. What made this an interesting find was that most people have to lose more weight than these study participants before seeing the same changes. It was a fascinating discovery which has spurred a significant number of individuals to try fasting.

Intermittent fasting for women has some beneficial effects. What makes it especially important for women who are trying to lose weight is that women have a much higher large proportion in their bodies. When trying to lose weight, the body primarily burns through carbohydrate stores with the first 6 hours and then starts to burn fat. Women who are following a healthy diet and exercise plan may be struggling with stubborn fat, but fasting is a realistic solution to this.

Intermittent Fasting For Women Over 50

Apparently, our bodies and our metabolism change when we hit menopause. One of the biggest changes that women over 50 experiences is that they have a slower metabolism and they start to put on weight. Fasting may be a good way to reverse and prevent this weight gain though. Studies have shown that this fasting pattern helps to regulate appetite and people who follow it regularly do not experience the same cravings that others do. If you're over 50 and trying to adjust to your slower metabolism, intermittent fasting can help you to avoid eating too much on a daily basis.

When you reach 50, your body also starts to develop some chronic diseases like high cholesterol and high blood pressure. Intermittent fasting has been shown to decrease both cholesterol and blood pressure, even without a large amount of weight loss. If you've started to notice your numbers rising at the doctor's office each year, you may be able to bring them back down with fasting, even without losing much weight.

Intermittent fasting may not be a splendid idea for every woman. Anyone with a particular health condition or who tends to be hypoglycemic should consult with a doctor. However, this new dietary trend has specific benefits for women who naturally store more fat in their bodies and may have trouble getting rid of these fat stores.

How To Quickly Lose Fat For Women

Losing fat can be very simple, but at the same time, it can be very frustrating. It's simple because weight loss is not a complicated equation. As long as you are consuming fewer calories than what your body burns you will lose weight. On the flipside, this can be very frustrating for those who don't know how to create the caloric deficit needed without depriving or starving themselves. Whatever the reason for wanting to lose weight, we are ultimately racing against time. So, here are the best ways to quickly lose fat for women.

Intermittent Fasting For Fat Loss

The fitness industry has given fasting for weight loss a bad rap over the past few years. There have been a lot of misconceptions and myths around fasting that people seem to get nervous about the idea. Let's first address the myths before we can move forward. Fasting does not cause your body to go into the infamous "starvation mode," nor does it slow the metabolism or breakdown muscle. The fitness industry has us believe that we have to regularly eat small meals throughout the day to keep the metabolism going. If we skip a meal or miss breakfast, our body goes into starvation mode which somehow causes the metabolism to slow down. It is one of the biggest myths in the industry.

The Wonderful Benefits Of Intermittent Fasting For Women

The pattern of eating called "Intermittent Fasting" usually means one fast for

a period and eats for a period. Many choose a 24-hour cycle of fasting, then eat healthy the next day, and continue this process as a lifestyle change.

Research has been done on animals to find the benefits of this type of fasting, and you will be happy to know it really can be beneficial to your health!

Intermittent fasting can add 40%-56% more years to your life! That in itself is reason enough to do it. However other benefits include body weight reduction and fat oxidation.

When you fast, your body is forced to scavenge for fuel thus removing aged and damaged cells in the process. It cleanses the body of annoying and unwanted things and helps the weight loss and benefits of the healthy food choices be increased and more beneficial to your body.

Rats have been shown to have long-term and improved survival after heart failure after being on an IF eating plan, too. Researchers are also saying that it might help age-related deficits in cognitive function, too, so that tells me that it might help ward off Alzheimer's Disease and other types of Dementia!

Your risk of heart disease and other heart ailments may also be decreased when you start a healthy intermittent fasting regimen. Your risk for other chronic illnesses and diseases will also most likely be reduced.

A healthier you can begin with intermittent fasting and healthy food choices! Keep carbs to 50-100 grams per day. Many women eat between 1200-1500 calories per day, and when limiting their carbs, they are still losing weight. Of course, less is best, and you need to determine caloric intake based on your activity such as working hard and exercising.

Drinking Lots Of Fluids

Drink lots of fluids, especially water and exercise in the evenings if possible. It will help with those late-night cravings.

Once you start eating and drinking healthier, your body won't crave as much (if any) junk food, so making healthy food choices will simply get easier and easier as you progress in the intermittent fasting routine.

Alternate Day Fasting or ADF means alternating days of eating and not eating any food, but there is also an intermittent fasting called Modified Fasting where you consume about 20% of your normal calories one day and then eat regularly (but healthy) the next day. It is often more attainable for people because they feel less deprived when they can at least eat something daily, and it still has most of the benefits of the ADF regimen.

Whatever you choose to do, make sure you tell your health care professional of your plans, so he or she is aware and can work with you to reach your goals. If you want to lose weight, lose fat and feel better, then intermittent fasting might be the answer for you!

To sum things up, you really can attain a feminine, firm, fit and younger appearance regardless of your age or inherited traits. You can overcome any weaknesses and trouble spots to some extent with balanced and symmetrical strength, cardiovascular and flexibility training, combined with making nutritious food choices.

Focus on being the best you can be. A lean and healthy body is both realistic and achievable.

Why Intermittent Fasting?

In the world today, there are numerous of ways that you can use to lose weight. But, why should you choose intermittent fasting over all those others?

This chapter is going to show you why intermittent fasting stands out among other weight loss methods by highlighting the various benefits that come with it as it is more than just a weight loss program. Some benefits you stand to gain by practicing intermittent fasting are as follows.

Better Detoxification

This may come to you as a surprise, but your body cleanses and detoxifies itself on a daily basis. Millions of cellular processes go on in your body, and it is usually your body's duty to identify the worn-out cells and replace them. This process is commonly known as autophagy, and it is a normal process that happens constantly.

The ongoing process of autophagy is usually affected by two things. The first one is a bad diet, and the second one is frequent eating. Usually, when you eat, the process of autophagy is slowed down because your body changes its focus from cleansing and detoxifying to digestion and absorption.

If you take meals only a few hours (5–6 hours) apart from each other, your cleansing process normally slows down making you feel tired as the lack of repair will be taking a toll on your cells.

One of the advantages of intermittent fasting is that it gives your body time to focus on the process of cellular repair because it discourages constant eating and encourages long hours of fasting. Therefore, with intermittent fasting, you stand a chance of boosting your body's detoxification process.

Less Hunger

Intermittent fasting is considered one of the best ways to lose weight because it deals with the one thing that makes it difficult for people to follow a diet, hunger.

Intermittent fasting is known for managing hunger and appetite, which makes the process of losing weight easier and fun. But how does it do this? Intense hunger is usually caused by blood sugar fluctuations, especially when your diet is high in carbohydrates.

When you eat a high-carb meal, your body produces high levels of insulin to manage the sugar levels. Insulin encourages your body cells to use the energy, and the rest is stored as fat, and this leads to a sudden drop in blood sugar levels. This sends a message to your brain that you need to eat to maintain your blood sugar level and the cycle continues.

Intermitted Fasting manages your appetite by controlling your hunger hormones. When you practice intermittent fasting, your body normally relies on stored fat for energy. When that happens, the fat cell produces a hormone called Leptin, which regulates the hunger hormone ghrelin. It does this by telling your brain to turn off the hunger signals from ghrelin, which makes you rarely feel hungry when you are fasting.

Lowered Risk of Type-2 Diabetes

One of the advantages of intermittent fasting is that it uses up all of the glucose in your body and starts using fat for energy. That process usually lowers your body's blood sugar levels, which in turn reduces your risk of getting type-2 diabetes.

According to a study that was done on intermittent fasting, it was found out that the blood sugar of a person practicing intermittent fasting reduced 3–6% while their insulin reduced by 20–31%. You can find this study here.

Reduced Oxidative Stress

Oxidative stress normally happens when your body has a higher production of free radicals than normal: free radicals include reactive oxygen species. Poorly functioning mitochondria normally cause These unstable molecules. Such molecules carry reactive electrons, which either take an electron or give up an electron when they encounter other molecules.

When that happens, the result is usually a fast chain reaction from one molecule to the other. That then ends up creating more of these free radicals that causes the connections between atoms in the DNA, cellular membrane, and the essential proteins to break apart and destroy. These damages not only stress your body out but also age you since your cells are constantly being damaged.

What intermittent fasting does is that it lowers your blood sugar levels, which automatically forces your cells to turn to a survival process. When this happens, the cells quickly remove any mitochondria that are unhealthy and substitute them with new ones that are healthy as time goes on. This activity is the one that reduces the production of free radicals, which translates to a reduction in oxidative stress.

Reduced Risk of Cancer

The relationship between intermittent fasting and cancer has been heavily debated upon up to date. Some people suggest that intermittent fasting reduces the risk of cancer while others believe that more research needs to be done. But if this research is anything to go by, then intermittent fasting can help you reduce the risk of cancer.

The study consisted of 10 cancer patients. Half of them were subjected to intermittent fasting before going for a chemotherapy session while the other half were not. After the two groups had gone for chemotherapy, it was discovered that the cancer patients who practiced intermittent fasting experienced reduced side effects and even had better cure rates than their counterparts did.

Cancer is usually caused by uncontrolled growth of cells, which mainly depend on the energy that comes from glucose to grow. Therefore, when you fast, you cut the energy channel that the cells need to grow. This causes the abnormal cells to stop growing completely or slow down.

Longevity

One of the most sort-after benefits of intermittent fasting is its ability to help you live a longer life. Numerous studies in rats have proven that intermittent fasting can extend your lifespan. In one of the rat studies, it was seen that rats that fasted daily lived 83% longer than those that didn't fast. Check out the study in the site below.

Now that you know how you can benefit from intermittent fasting, the next step is for you to find out how you can start practicing intermittent fasting and the methods that you will be using.

Types of Intermittent Fasting

Intermittent fasting has become very trendy in the past few years, and several different types/methods have emerged.

Here are some of the most popular ones:

- **The 16/8 Method**: Fast for 16 hours each day, for example by only eating between noon and 8pm.
- **Eat-Stop-Eat**: Once or twice a week, don't eat anything from dinner one day, until dinner the next day (a 24 hour fast).
- **The 5:2 Diet**: During 2 days of the week, eat only about 500-600 calories.

Then there are many other variations.

I am personally a fan of the 16/8 method (popularized by Martin Berkhan of LeanGains), as I find it to be the simplest and the easiest to stick to.

In fact, I pretty much naturally eat this way. I am usually not very hungry in the morning, and don't feel compelled to eat until about 1 pm.

Then I eat my last meal somewhere between 6-9pm, so I end up instinctively fasting for 16-19 hours every day.

Bottom Line: There are many different intermittent fasting methods. The most popular ones are the 16/8 method, Eat-Stop-Eat and the 5:2 diet.

Take Home Message

As long as you stick to healthy foods, restricting your eating window and fasting from time to time can have some very impressive health benefits.

It is an effective way to lose fat and improve metabolic health, while simplifying your life at the same time.

Popular Ways to do Intermittent Fasting

1. The 16/8 Method: Fast for 16 hours each day

The 16/8 Method involves fasting every day for 14-16 hours, and restricting your daily "eating window" to 8-10 hours. Within the eating window, you can fit in 2, 3 or more meals.

This method is also known as the Leangains protocol, and was popularized by fitness expert Martin Berkhan. Doing this method of fasting can actually be as simple as not eating anything after dinner, and skipping breakfast.

For example, if you finish your last meal at 8 pm and then don't eat until 12 noon the next day, then you are technically fasting for 16 hours between meals.

It is generally recommended that women only fast 14-15 hours, because they seem to do better with slightly shorter fasts. For people who get hungry in the morning and like to eat breakfast, then this can be hard to get used to at first. However, many breakfast skippers actually instinctively eat this way. You can drink water, coffee and other non-caloric beverages during the fast, and this can help reduce hunger levels.

It is very important to eat mostly healthy foods during your eating window. This won't work if you eat lots of junk food or excessive amounts of calories.

I find this to be the most "natural" way to do intermittent fasting. I eat this way myself and find it to be 100% effortless.

I eat a low-carb diet, so my appetite is blunted somewhat. I simply do not feel hungry until around 1 pm in the afternoon. Then I eat my last meal around 6-9 pm, so I end up fasting for 16-19 hours.

Bottom Line: The 16/8 method involves daily fasts of 16 hours for men, and 14-15 hours for women. On each day, you restrict your eating to an

8-10 hour "eating window" where you can fit in 2-3 or more meals.

2. The 5:2 Diet: Fast for 2 days per week.

The 5:2 diet involves eating normally 5 days of the week, while restricting calories to 500-600 on two days of the week. This diet is also called the Fast diet, and was popularized by British journalist and doctor Michael Mosley. On the fasting days, it is recommended that women eat 500 calories, and men 600 calories.

For example, you might eat normally on all days except Mondays and Thursdays, where you eat two small meals (250 calories per meal for women, and 300 for men). As critics correctly point out, there are no studies testing the 5:2 diet itself, but there are plenty of studies on the benefits of intermittent fasting.

Bottom Line: The 5:2 diet, or the Fast diet, involves eating 500-600 calories for two days of the week but eating normally the other 5 days.

3. Eat-Stop-Eat: Do a 24-hour fast, once or twice a week.

Eat-Stop-Eat involves a 24-hour fast, either once or twice per week. This method was popularized by fitness expert Brad Pilon, and has been quite popular for a few years.

By fasting from dinner one day, to dinner the next, this amounts to a 24-hour fast.

For example, if you finish dinner on Monday at 7 pm, and don't eat until dinner the next day at 7 pm, then you've just done a full 24-hour fast. You can also fast from breakfast to breakfast, or lunch to lunch. The end result is the same. Water, coffee and other non-caloric beverages are allowed during the fast, but no solid food.

If you are doing this to lose weight, then it is very important that you eat normally during the eating periods. As in, eat the same amount of food as if you hadn't been fasting at all.

The problem with this method is that a full 24-hour fast can be fairly difficult for many people.

However, you don't need to go all-in right away, starting with 14-16 hours and then moving upwards from there is fine. I've personally done this a few times. I found the first part of the fast very easy, but in the last few hours I did become ravenously hungry.

I needed to apply some serious self-discipline to finish the full 24-hours and often found myself giving up and eating dinner a bit earlier.

Bottom Line: Eat-Stop-Eat is an intermittent fasting program with one or two 24-hour fasts per week.

4. Alternate-Day Fasting: Fast every other day.

Alternate-Day fasting means fasting every other day. There are several different versions of this. Some of them allow about 500 calories during the fasting days. Many of the lab studies showing health benefits of intermittent fasting used some version of this. A full fast every other day seems rather extreme, so I do not recommend this for beginners. With this method, you will be going to bed very hungry several times per week, which is not very pleasant and probably unsustainable in the long-term.

Bottom Line: Alternate-day fasting means fasting every other day, either by not eating anything or only eating a few hundred calories.

5. The Warrior Diet: Fast during the day, eat a huge meal at night.

The Warrior Diet was popularized by fitness expert Ori Hofmekler. It involves eating small amounts of raw fruits and vegetables during the day, then eating one huge meal at night.

Basically, you "fast" all day and "feast" at night within a 4 hour eating window. The Warrior Diet was one of the first popular "diets" to include a form of intermittent fasting. This diet also emphasizes food choices that are quite similar to a paleo diet – whole, unprocessed foods that resemble what they looked like in nature.

Bottom Line: The Warrior Diet is about eating only small amounts of vegetables and fruits during the day, then eating one huge meal at night.

6. Spontaneous Meal Skipping: Skip meals when convenient.

You don't need to follow a structured intermittent fasting plan to reap some of the benefits. Another option is to simply skip meals from time to time, when you don't feel hungry or are too busy to cook and eat. It is a myth that people need to eat every few hours, or they will hit "starvation mode" or lose muscle. The human body is well equipped to handle long periods of famine, let alone missing one or two meals from time to time.

So if you're not hungry one day, skip breakfast and just eat a healthy lunch and dinner. Or if you're travelling somewhere and can't find anything you want to eat, do a short fast.

Skipping 1 or 2 meals when you feel so inclined is basically a spontaneous intermittent fast. Just make sure to eat healthy foods at the other meals.

Bottom Line: Another more "natural" way to do intermittent fasting is to simply skip 1 or 2 meals when you don't feel hungry or don't have time to eat.

Take Home Message

There are a lot of people getting great results with some of these methods.

That being said, if you're already happy with your health and don't see much room for improvement, then feel free to safely ignore all of this. Intermittent fasting is not for everyone. It is not something that anyone needs to do, it is just another tool in the toolbox that can be useful for some people. Some also believe that it may not be as beneficial for women as men, and it may also be a poor choice for people who are prone to eating disorders. If you decide to try this out, then keep in mind that you need to eat healthy as well. It is not possible to binge on junk foods during the eating periods and expect to lose weight and improve health.

Calories still count, and foodquality is still absolutely crucial.

Specific Considerations When Implementing Intermittent Fasting

You've now got a thorough understanding of the background of intermittent fasting, the scientifically based evidence of its benefits, how to do it, and how to work this cycle of eating into your life.

There are some considerations as to who may or may not benefit from intermittent fasting. There are a lot of women (and men) who have gotten great weight loss results using some form of fasting and cycled eating. However, just like any diet and exercise program or regimen, intermittent fasting is not for everyone, and it's important you practice the proper weight loss plan for your body and your specific goals. Intermittent fasting is certainly not something that everyone needs to do, but it's a helpful tool in the weight loss battle that so many women struggle with. It can be easily implemented in many women's daily lives and used to promote greater overall health and well-being, but it can, in some cases, be misused as well.

There are a few pre-requisites that if followed, will make your intermittent fasting weight loss journey easier and more successful, and make you a good candidate for reaping the most benefits from this program. These include the following:

- Get enough sleep on a regular basis.

- Minimize stress in your daily life.

- Make sure lifestyle activity is within a normal range—not too much or too little daily movement and/or exercise.

- Be fat adapted. This means that your body can easily access and burn stored fat throughout the day when it's needed to provide energy.

So, how can you tell if you're already considered fat adapted? No blood test can give you this answer, but there are a few simple questions you can ask yourself that should be able to provide you with an indication of your level of fat adaptability:

• Can you go 3 hours or more without eating? Would skipping a meal be an incredibly difficult physical and mental struggle for you?

• On a normal day, do you feel your energy level stays consistent throughout the day? Do you need to take an afternoon nap or is it just something you enjoy doing now and again?

• Are you able to perform fairly vigorous physical activity like steady walking, jogging, or light exercise without first consuming carbohydrates for energy?

• Do you frequently suffer from headaches, mental exhaustion, and mental fog?

Someone whose body is fat adapted can usually skip meals with little effort on their part. They have consistent energy and do not require an afternoon nap to make it through the second portion of their day. They are able to be moderately active and perform physical activities like brisk walking, jogging, hiking, biking, and swimming without needing to fuel their body beforehand with carbohydrates, and they do not suffer from the mental fog, headaches, and exhaustion that a person whose body is more sugar dependent may.

Some of you are lucky and are genetically predisposed to be a fat burning machine! Others of you may not be, and your genetics may require more effort than the first group to reach this state of fat burning and freedom from sugar and carbohydrate dependence. Luckily for all of us, your genes are not final! They don't define you, and they can be altered! Through your behavior and your lifestyle choices, you have the ability to turn on and off various genes in your genetic code that can lead to the physical results you desire. There are numerous versions of the future person you may become, and it's always up to you to make the decisions that will ultimately lead to who you will become. You are responsible for making choices and living a lifestyle that will promote and direct your genes toward fat loss, building muscle, and overall wellness. Following an intermittent fasting style of eating will put you on the path to achieving this longevity of life and general wellness of the body.

If you feel that you may be lacking in the fat-adaptability department and want to give yourself the best start to your intermittent fasting protocol, it can benefit you to try eating the paleo style diet for 3 weeks before beginning your cycles of fasting and eating. This basically means you'll eliminate sugar, grains, legumes, and vegetable oils from your diet for 3 weeks prior to beginning intermittent fasting. This should be the push your body needs to become more efficient in drawing upon fat stores for energy rather than relying on dietary sugar for fuel. Again, this step is not necessary for your pursuit of weight loss through intermittent fasting, but it can set you up for the most success in the shortest amount of time.

Are there any indicators of someone whom intermittent fasting may not be beneficial for?

Intermittent fasting may not be a great protocol to follow for someone who is susceptible to eating disorders. If you've had a problem with disordered eating at any point in your life, it might be beneficial for you to explore multiple weight loss plans before deciding what works best for you. If intermittent fasting seems like the best choice for your lifestyle, do take the time to pay special attention to the amount of food you're consuming when you are not in your fasting periods, just to be sure you do not continuously deny yourself nutrition.

Intermittent fasting is considered a stressor on your body systems. You're using planned fasting and hunger to ignite metabolic processes within your body that respond to these stressors. For this reason, someone with a multitude of other stressors may not fare as well while following an intermittent fasting protocol. Mental stress, physical stress, and emotional stress can all hinder your mental ability to properly complete your fasting cycles as well as your body's physical ability to lose weight. Adding this new stressor can compound any other existing stressors, which won't be the most effective way to begin your weight loss journey.

Intermittent fasting may not be beneficial for someone with a cortisol regulation disorder. If you're actively monitoring your cortisol levels with your doctor or if you think you may have an issue with cortisol regulation it would be best to seek a professional opinion before implementing a fast into your weight loss regimen. Fasting raises cortisol levels in the body, and in a healthy individual, this poses no threat or health issue. Someone with a cortisol dysregulation can have serious side effects if their levels become excessive, and an activity that boosts production of cortisol may not be right for these people. If you think you may have an issue with cortisol regulation, visit your doctor before starting a program and find out for sure. You may have an issue with cortisol regulation if you retain excess belly fat, consistently lack enough sleep, persistently suffer from low-grade stress, and rely on caffeine to keep you awake and energized each day.

Should a pregnant woman practice intermittent fasting?

There haven't been many studies done on the effects of fasting on pregnant women on their growing fetus. One study17 that followed pregnant women fasting for Ramadan showed that these women had a decrease in the development and growth of their placentas, but the slower growth was more efficient. The developing fetus grew as normal, but the women had much smaller reserves of nutrients in their bodies. Although this (and a few other) studies show that short-term fasting is probably safe during pregnancy, it is most likely a better idea to wait until after giving birth. Fasting during pregnancy is not necessary (except in these cases of religiously required fasts) and is probably not beneficial to the woman or her growing baby.

Should I fast if I am a diabetic?

This is a gray area and should be reviewed with your doctor before you begin. Women have a more difficult time regulating their blood sugar than men and can be more severely affected by a drop in blood sugar. There have been accounts of men who were classified as diabetic using intermittent fasting to control their blood sugar levels, lose weight, and effectively beat type-2 diabetes, but there have been no such accounts for women.

Will intermittent fasting affect my menstrual cycle and fertility?

Humans are highly biologically effective at adapting to their environments. When proper nutrition is not available, it is more work for a woman's body to create new life and provide nutrition for the baby once it's born. For this reason, women are biologically designed to respond to the presence or scarcity of available food by altering some aspects of fertility. There haven't been clinical studies directly comparing the effects of intermittent fasting on female fertility. These studies do have to look at, mostly, and compare fertility changes due to extreme fasting circumstances like famine or anorexia—which are not truly comparable to planned and purposeful intermittent fasting. These studies do show a link between decreased fertility, the loss of a menstrual cycle, and fasting, but the differences between these scenarios and intermittent fasting should be considered. There is currently too little evidence-based clinical information on the relationship between intermittent fasting and female

49

reproductive health to definitively say if it is beneficial, neutral, or harmful.

Do I Need To Change My Diet If I Use Intermittent Fasting?

I will begin by saying again that you should eat as healthily as you can – less processed junk, whole foods and plenty of green vegetables and water. However, you can be less than perfect with nutrition and still achieve results while fasting. It can be especially helpful to binge a little to keep sane – especially when trying something as demanding as fasting. Just don't consume more calories than you burn.

Onto the point though - intermittent fasting itself never requires a diet change by definition. Only a change in the times that you allow yourself to eat is necessary. Whether or not you choose to change your diet is up to you. Some people use IF purely for its health benefits. Others use it to prevent heart disease and diabetes. If you plan to lose weight and burn fat, however, you will need to change your diet in conjunction with IF.

The formula for weight loss is incredibly simple - so simple that it sounds almost too good to be true. All you need to do is take in less energy (calories) than you expend. That's it. It may sound easy, but in reality, it can be tough. Any health guru or fitness god who tells you that there's an easier way is quite simply lying and trying to sell you something. Sure, fat and nutrient macros are necessary if you are looking to maximize results and want a specific body fat percentage or maybe even if you're a bodybuilder. But if all you want to do is lose weight, energy (calories) is the only thing that matters. This is where IF comes in. Let's think of this mathematically.

To calculate how much energy (calories) you naturally spend without any exercise, you can use this formula:

655 + (4.35 × weight in lbs) + (4.7 × height in inches) − (4.7 × age)

If you are a 200 pound, 5' 5", 27-year-old woman and you use Alternate Day Fasting (ADF)...

You expend 1,703 calories a day naturally, or 11,925 a week.

You take in 400 calories on your non-feeding days.

You take in 2,000 calories on your feeding days.

You take in 9,200 calories per week total.

That leaves an energy (calorie) deficit of 2,725 calories. A pound of fat is about 3,500 calories. That's almost a pound of fat lost per week with no exercise, and probably without even changing your eating habits that much on feeding days. You can imagine how much more you'd lose by eating a bit healthier and exercising on your non-feeding days.

If you are using IF without a diet change, you'll still reap significant health benefits, but results won't be the absolute best. However, that doesn't mean that you can eat pizza and cake on every feeding day. If you're a regular Sally and you eat sensibly, to begin with, your diet doesn't have to change dramatically. High-fat and low-fat diets have no effect on the health benefits of IF. This is one of the many reasons that IF is so popular these days. It's a simple, proven method for improving your health and extending your lifespan.

The Lessons You Learn While Intermittent Fasting

Intermittent fasters have reported improved strength and leaner figures. The best part of this is that they didn't give up their favorite foods and feel cranky like they would have otherwise. While fasting, these same people have learned all sorts of lessons about the fasting process. They might provide a helpful guide to anyone that's getting started on the journey of intermittent fasting.

The biggest roadblock is your mind.

This diet, in comparison to all the other ones out there, is quite simple to implement into your life. Depending on how you have set up your fasting, you skip certain meals and make up for them at other meals. The biggest hurdle in this is telling your mind to accept the changes. People believe that if they aren't eating at particular times, they're going to faint or become ill or have some other adverse effects. People also believe that these particular times are roughly a couple hours apart. They also believe that skipping breakfast will ruin your day or that a light dinner will make them hungry during the night.

Starting fasting will help you realize how simple the diet is. People feel much healthier inside and out when they practice fasting. Many people find it best to ease into the diet instead of jumping in all at once. The lifestyle can go against everything that you were taught as children. You may even feel that it is adversely affecting your health to do something like this. However, you will see how wrong you were once you see intermittent fasting in action.

Over time, you will find that your fears have no basis in the reality of the situation. You'll be healthier and more energetic than you were before you started intermittent fasting. The only thing you need to do is get yourself started on this journey.

You can easily lose weight and keep it off.

When you're consuming less calories than you burn, you lose weight. That's how weight lose works. Intermittent fasting is an easy method to this because it also avoids losing muscle mass. Those who need to lose weight for health reasons may turn to intermittent fasting because it doesn't mean much of a change in the diet that they had before intermittent fasting. The only change is when eating happens. Intermittent fasting works because when you eliminate meals and eat during your feeding time, there is a deficit of calories, assuming you don't completely binge.

Building muscle while fasting is extremely possible.

While using intermittent fasting, people report being able to gain lean muscle and cut off the fat by five percent. During the fasting period, your body is likely to lose weight. Because there is no steady flow of food and energy, your body will learn to turn to your fat stores and pull energy from there instead.

Because the fasts are short enough, your body won't turn to cannibalizing the muscles for energy. This means that there's little risk of losing muscle mass while practicing intermittent fasting. With eating, as long as you're consuming enough calories to build muscle, your body doesn't care when that food consumption happens. If it happens during an 8-hour period, the calories will affect you roughly the same as if you had eaten those calories over a 16-hour period or a 24-hour period.

Intermittent fasting can help your productivity.

While practicing intermittent fasting, many people report having improved metal clarity. This is especially true during the fasting periods. While we are told that fasting drains the body and mind of energy, this just simply true. When the mind isn't focused so much on food, it can free up time for you to think about your other interests and hobbies.

Instead of thinking about dinner, you can think about a project that you've wanted to work on for a while. There's less time wasted when you're making even one less meal a day. You don't have to shop, cook, wash, or spend time eating for that extra meal. You also don't have to worry about everything involved in it. The freed up time, and mental energy is great for getting on with projects and things that you want to get involved in.

Change up your foods on a regular basis.

When you're using intermittent fasting, you want to rotate your foods and calories according to your schedule. On the days that you're working out, you'll want to eat a little bit more. On the days that you're resting, you'll want to reduce the calories that you're consuming. This will help balance out the calories so that you're building muscles when you're working out and burning fat while you're not working out. Cutting down a little on rest days should be easy since you won't need the extra calories. It will be a mental workout instead of a physical one. During those rest days, you'll be going through more of your fat stores than otherwise.

However, besides the calorie counts, you need to make sure that you're also looking at the nutrients that you're eating. More protein on days that you're working out will help you a lot. When you're taking it easy, you'll need a slightly different nutrient set. If you keep changing up your carbs and protein by when you're working out and resting, then you'll find yourself becoming a leaner, fit person quite quickly.

There are no shortcuts when it comes to dieting and fasting.

When people hear stories about losing tons of weight in a short amount of time, they get excited about the diet. When they try it, and it doesn't work in a week, they feel disappointed and often give up. The short term view of dieting and fasting gets in the way of actually losing weight. Instead of thinking about the seven days in a week individually, you would do better to focus on the longer term and think about what you're eating over the course of a week. Instead of micromanaging your hours, focus on the day as a whole and getting the nutrients in at some point during the day.

Your body won't care about when the nutrients get into your body. Whether it's a protein shake one hour or twelve hours later, your body will still get the protein. You just need to ensure that you are getting the calories and nutrients necessary for your health and fitness. You're just shifting when exactly those get to your body in an intermittent fasting schedule. If you focus on the longer term, you'll realize that ultimately fasting will do you good.

When fasting, you will want less food.

On a fast, you slowly pull away from the restraints of your food addictions and diet. You'll be eating because you want to, not because you are on a schedule that dictates when you will eat. This change won't be obvious at first. It may take weeks or months or maybe even a year before you're free from those cravings that you used to have. As time passes, you'll feel more comfortable fasting. You won't crave food as you did before. You may even develop a better appreciation for food when you do eat. Your mind will think of eating as something other than the chore that it is when you're not on an intermittent fast. It will be an extremely enjoyable time, instead of just something that you have to do.

Losing fat and building muscle doesn't happen at the same time.

If you're looking to not only lose fat but also gain muscle, then you'll have to do some specific things with your intermittent fasting to get it to work with you. You'll have to use calorie cycling as well to help you get to the gains and losses that you want in your body. To lose weight, you'll need to be taking in less calories than you're burning off. But for muscle gain, you'll need to have enough calories and nutrients to help your muscles along. So the two processes are already at odds because you can't have a calorie deficit for weight loss and a calorie surplus for muscle gain at the same time.

If you consider longer time frames, you might begin to see how the two working together can make you a better you.

You will get a better result if you train a little less while fasting.

When you're fasting, you should consider a long-term when you look at your training. Instead of daily goals, pick out goals for the week's workout sessions. Once you've decided that, make sure that you're doing the most important and effective exercises first. Doing compound exercises early will help you get the most out of your fast. You may decide on the way to split the workout through the day. You could use the upper body in the morning and lower body in the afternoon. It could look more like pushups in the morning and squats in the afternoon.

Your workouts will be much more effective during a fast because of the changes going on in your body. Both hormonal and metabolic changes are happening. These changes will mean that you'll need less training to get the same amount of change. Intermittent fasting will allow your body to change more quickly and more efficiently. Less time will mean that you've got more time to pursue other goals. It's a win for you in every way.

Drinking a lot of water will help you throughout fasting.

One of the most important things to remember while using intermittent fasting is that you need to keep yourself hydrated. Your needs may be different than someone else, but the general rule is to drink around two liters of water every day. You may not feel like you want to or need it, but you should do it anyways. Your body will only tell you that it's thirty when it is dehydrated. This is something to be avoided.

Humans obtain some of our water from the foods we consume. There are some foods, like vegetables, which are more efficient at providing water content. Because you will be eating less, you won't be getting an extra water boost throughout the day. Drinking water often will help counter the loss.

Water may also help you battle hunger pains during the day. It'll help you conquer the mental battle not to eat all the time. There aren't many problems that can come from drinking water, so you should consume lots of it to help with the intermittent fast that you're on. Other liquids are allowed, but water will be the most beneficial to them all.

The best diet is the one that works for your body.

Everyone wants the easy road to the best possible life. They want it to be something that will dramatically change them quick. Diet books sell like crazy because people are always looking for that one thing that will improve their lives so much. A quick fix is what they're looking for. However, the quick fix rarely works. Everyone is slightly different, and diets will affect them differently. Not all diets will take into account every single thing, like gender, age, body type, fitness levels, medical conditions, or allergies. All of these things, and more contribute to how your body works. You won't be able to follow a quick fix probably because of these reasons. To find what works for your body, you're going to need some time and patience to experiment and see what works best.

Intermittent fasting does well in this regard. While using this method for weight loss, you can experiment with how your eating schedule and patterns are set up. This experimentation won't cause harm to your body and health. As you experiment, there will be foods and eating schedules that make you feel full of energy and ones that make you feel lethargic or otherwise unhealthy. As you figure out what is and isn't working, you'll be slowly tweaking your life to make it into a better one. This is one of the reasons why intermittent fasting is so much better than most other diets. You're not restricted to the foods you eat, just the amount of time that you have to eat.

Exercise and Intermittent Fasting

One common question people have when doing intermittent fasting is whether or not it is safe and healthy to exercise either aerobically or anaerobically while they are, say, "running on empty" freak out the Jackson Browne! But, if done correctly, the combination can help you burn lots your body's fat reserves quickly. Maintaining some exercise routine is vital for your mental and physical health – that's a given. So, in fact, exercising and running in a fasted state is an excellent way to become fat adapted and improve your mental state at the same time.

You've already heard the adage, 80% diet, 20% exercise – to combine dieting with exercise. This is true! Imagine if we could make our body burn more fat for fuel while at rest, and then also burn fat more efficiently during exercise. Most of us have 40,000 calories of fat in our bodies at any given time and around 1,200 calories of muscle glycogen or sugar. Imagine how far or how much we could exercise if we had access to that 40,000-calorie fuel tank. That's 33 times the amount of energy fuel! So, perhaps next time you run out of energy in the middle of an exercise routine, you will wish your body was in fat-burning mode instead of calorie-burning mode.

The first step to burning more fat during exercise is: you need to have what's called an "aerobic base." The way to build this base is thru aerobic heart rate training, which will raise what is known as your "aerobic capacity." Aerobic capacity is defined as the maximal amount of oxygen in milliliters (ml) that an athlete utilizes in one minute, per kilogram of body weight. In layman's terms, the higher the "aerobic base" or "capacity," the more body work you can do in one minute. The best method I have found for heart rate training is Phil Maffetone's "MAF" training.

What does this mean for exercise? Technically, by having a higher aerobic base, we boost the size and strength of our heart, the concentration of hemoglobin in our blood, the density of our capillaries, and the number of mitochondria in our muscles. The benefits expand beyond the scope of this book, but essentially by developing an aerobic base, we become healthier inside and out.

What this means for intermittent fasting is that when you are training in a fasted state, your body becomes superbly efficient at burning fat for fuel. From an aerobic aspect your body can more efficiently utilize oxygen and this, in turn, makes you more efficient at exercise aerobically or anaerobically. You must first develop your aerobic base to enhance anaerobic exercise.

If you are looking to add muscle, fasting can help by increasing the production of certain hormones in your body. Other than weight training and getting the proper amount of sleep regularly, fasting has proven to be one of the most effective methods of increasing human growth hormone, or "HGH." Studies have also suggested that fasting in combination with regular exercise can increase the levels of testosterone in men and women, which is another hormone that can decrease body fat and increase muscle mass. Here are my recommendations for adding muscle:

• Don't push yourself too hard. If you are doing "cardio" exercise, as a test, make sure you can carry on a conversation at the same time; otherwise, you may be pushing yourself too hard. When you are doing the exercise slowly, but for a long time, that's when your body is becoming more "fat adapted." That's when it is going into a ketogenic state. Listen always to your body, and stop if you start to feel dizzy or lightheaded.

• The 16/8 method, in particular, recommends scheduling your meals for when you plan to finish doing any moderate-to-intense exercise. Plan your high-intensity workouts for around a time when you are getting ready to break your fast so that you can eat soon thereafter. Properly scheduled, if your workout is very intense, you can follow it with a carbohydrate-rich snack.

- If you are lifting weights, make sure you are getting adequate protein or supplementing with adequate BCAAs. "Feast" on meals that are high in protein. Eating protein on a regular basis is vital to muscle growth.
- When planning your meals with workouts in mind, try combining fast-acting simple carbohydrates with a protein that will serve to stabilize your blood sugar after your workout. A banana and some peanut butter is a good example.

Here are some sample routines for nourishment while exercising when using intermittent fasting:

Early Morning Exercise:

- Exercise fasted in the early morning: aerobic or anaerobic. Examples: running or weights
- Take BCAAs afterward - up to 30 grams before lunch.
- Around Noon: Eat lunch. Aim for about 20-25% of your daily calorie intake.
- Around 3 PM: Snack on high-fat foods, nuts, and seeds.
- Between 4-5 PM: Eat dinner. This should be your largest meal of the day.
- Fast from 8 pm until noon the next day.

Lunch Time Exercise:

- Just before Noon: Take up to 30 grams of BCAAs.

- Exercise fasted at lunch: aerobic or anaerobic. Again as examples: running, or weights
- After exercising around 1-2pm: Eat lunch. Aim for 20-25% of your daily calorie intake.
- Around 3-4 PM: Snack on high-fat foods, nuts, and seeds
- Around 6 PM: Eat dinner. This meal's calories should approximate your lunch's.
- Around 8-9 PM: Eat something light. Snack if needed.
- Fast from 9 pm or 10 pm until 1-2pm the next day.

You will likely not be working out every single day. So, on rest days, your biggest meal of the day should be your first one instead of your last. On rest days, aim for consuming roughly 35-40% of your calories in your first meal, and eat a lot of protein and fat as part of this meal.

Common Mistakes When Fasting

You still eat unhealthy foods

If you are eating McDonalds every day as a part of your daily meal or meals – depending on which plan you pick – then you have your work cut out for you. You need to switch to unprocessed healthy foods for maximum impact. Try to consume a large meal of wild meat or organic vegetables and see the difference.

This principle extends to beverages too. Stick to water, unsweetened coffee or tea and cut out all the processed juices and carbonated beverages from your diet.

You do not stay busy

Every time someone tells you "hey here is a secret for you to keep" your basic instinct is to go around and tell everyone! Similarly, when you are told, "do not eat food" your unconscious urge is to go and eat everything that you can!

So, when you are fasting, go and find something to do. Go golfing or take a swim. Read a book or watch your favorite show on Netflix (not Master Chef though!) anything to keep you distracted and occupied. Avoid going places where there is bound to be food.

You have too many stimulants

Intermittent Fasting allows you to switch your breakfast for a cup or two of unsweetened coffee. The caffeine keeps you alert, and the coffee fills you up a bit, helping you to feel full for a while. A few cups of coffee before lunch is fine, but don't get addicted to it to the extent that it starts replacing food.

You start out over ambitious

Do not start your Intermittent Fasting journey by directly jumping in with 24-hour fasting; you are just setting yourself up for failure. When you switch from frequently eating to not eating at all (or eating a single meal), it is too severe a change for your body to adjust to. Start out with the 16/8 diet initially, then slowly add in a day of Eat Stop Eat once a week and then shift to a meal a day diet. The slow progression will help your body to adjust to the change, and it will be easier for you.

You are scared of feeling hungry

Feeling hungry is a normal bodily reaction. It doesn't mean that you are starving or your bodily functions will stop, or you will die. Your body is made of a lot of tougher stuff and can easily handle fasting periods of 16 or 20 hours. So do not feel scared, it is just a reaction, and if you ignore it, the pangs will go away.

More is not better

Wow! After fasting for 24 hours I felt so good, why don't I fast for 481 hours? Or even for 72 hours? Well, the benefits of fasting start reducing after a fasting period of 20 hours. There is a thin but firm line that separates fasting from starving, do not cross it!

You are not accepting the chaos

When you make your nutrition consumption schedule a little haphazard, your body goes into a state of chaos and in this state of chaos, whenever you consume anything; the body immediately absorbs all the required nutrients as it is unsure when the next feeding will be. So, Intermittent Fasting provides your body with stress that it needs to learn to cope with slowly and this short-term deprivation just makes your body more efficient. So, when you accept this chaos, you make your body work in a more efficient manner.

You are continuously looking at the clock

You are a human and not a machine. You do not need to do things by the hands of a clock. Eat when you are ready to eat, not when the clock tells you to. If you are very hungry and it is not the time for your meal, munch on a few raw fruits or vegetables. Do not look at the clock but just say it is not dinner time and continue to keep yourself going. Your feeding window is a rough time frame, not an absolute compulsion.

Tips to Stay Motivated

Have you managed to shed some weight? And then regain whatever you have managed to shed? Well, it isn't a rocket science to figure it out that you were low on motivation. But then a few weeks into it your motivation starts to falter? Well, don't worry. This is normal. It happens to the best of us. Having the same old boring meals might leave you feeling frustrated and annoyed. You might end up binging on things you have been avoiding for so long. A few slip-ups and you feel emotionally as well as physically derailed. Don't let this get to you. Having the right motivation can help you stick to a diet without having to worry about any distractions. Attitude matters as much as keeping an eye on what you eat and how much you exercise. All your efforts will go for a toss if you don't stay motivated. Going through the process of weight loss will take time, and it does get difficult especially with all the temptations that we are surrounded with.

Set realistic goals

The first thing you need to do while wanting to diet is set goals. You need to be able to maintain your mojo throughout the process and not just during the initial few weeks. One of the factors that have a major impact on whether or not your diet will prove to be a success is the goals you set for yourself. If you are setting goals that are simply unattainable, then you are just setting yourself up for failure. If you set the goal of losing 30 pounds in a month, then that's physically impossible and dangerous as well. Set goals that are attainable. You can set long-term as well as short-term goals. Your short-term goal can be shedding 5 pounds in one month. That's perfectly achievable, and when you achieve the goal you have set for yourself, the chances of you succeeding again are high.

Expect setbacks

You need to understand that it is okay to experience setbacks. A setback isn't a failure it simply means a delay. And every one of us cannot resist temptation every single time. There will be times when you won't be able to resist temptation, and you might give in. The danger isn't about eating something once, but it shouldn't become an excuse for you to binge every single time. Don't think that just because you have gone off track once, you will do it again. Just accept your mistake and ensure that you don't repeat it ever again.

Don't try to be a perfectionist

So, you have managed to gobble down a pint of ice cream or had a cheeseburger for lunch? Don't try to be a perfectionist here. Perfectionist thinking hinders success. If you indulge in a 200-calorie treat, then it is all right and perfectly normal. You are human after all. But this cannot be the reason for giving into a 1000-calorie indulgence just because you have broken your diet once. If you do slip up, you need to remember that it is perfectly all right. Everyone has their moments once in a while. You need to remember that you should keep going and don't give up.

Buddy system is helpful

It is difficult when you are swimming upstream, especially when you are doing everything all by yourself. It might be really helpful if you have someone else who has got similar goals. Your buddy will provide the support system that you require and will also keep you in check every time you are going off course. It might be really difficult to resist temptation, and when you have someone else by your side who is in the same position as you are, then it will work wonders for yourself confidence. There are various support groups out there that can help you with this.

You will need to be patient

Don't expect any results to happen overnight. The journey of shedding weight will take some time. You will need to be patient. You cannot expect miracles. You will need to follow your diet closely. You will need to exercise regularly and eat right. It will take a while for your efforts to pay off. But they will pay off, and when they do, you will be pleasantly surprised. It is all right even if the results don't show after a week. You will need to stay on track. You can make changes to your diet plan if you think a particular diet isn't working. Just see to it that you aren't going back to your unhealthy ways.

Remember to reward yourself

You need to remember to reward yourself every time you do something right. You can criticize yourself when you do something wrong, but you should also reward yourself whenever you do something right. It needn't be anything expensive.

Maybe you can treat yourself to a day out at a spa or probably buy yourself that pair of shoes you have wanted forever. But don't reward yourself with those foods that you aren't supposed to eat. You can set short-term as well as long-term goals and reward yourself whenever you achieve any of your goals.

You will need a maintenance plan

It is an achievement that you have managed to achieve your goal. But your work isn't done, yet. You will need to develop a maintenance plan that will help you ensure that the weight that you have managed to shed keeps off. It is not just about attaining your physical goal, but it is also about maintaining it. You will need to devise a plan that will help you stay on track even in the long run. But it needn't be as strict as your diet plan. For making a plan, you can always consult an expert so that you get the guidance you need.

So, you will need to do everything that you can for staying motivated. Your efforts will pay off. Always remember to keep a positive outlook. Don't let any negativity make you doubt yourself.

Conclusion

If you want to stick to intermittent fasting for life, then you must not view it as a diet but as a lifestyle. This will require you to re-evaluate your eating choices even before beginning the fast so that when you begin, you are sure that you won't be going back. For example, if you use regular vegetable oil then it is time to replace it with healthy oils such as coconut oil and olive oil. If you tend to eat processed carbs, then it is time to replace them with healthy whole, unprocessed carbs- e.g. zucchini noodles in place of pasta.

The idea here is to embrace the diet and the fact that your body will be a full on fat burning means that new carbs won't be required for body fuel. It will typically take a few weeks for this to happen but once it does, cravings for unhealthy carbs will be out of the picture and incorporating this diet into your life will be as easy as ABC.

If you are going to live the ultimate intermittent fasting lifestyle, then:

The best way to include Intermittent Fasting into your lifestyle is by delaying your breakfast slowly by slowly- delay by an hour then another hour the next day and so on. Take an hour to shower, an hour to do your chores, an hour to get to work- just take an hour from any activity that you engage in the morning that you see the best fit until you get to a time that you can live with.

Do not use fasting as an excuse to eat junk- calories are different. 100 calories of broccoli are not the same as 100 calories of a snicker bar. When you find yourself cheating then get real with yourself. Keep the carbs for before workouts and fill yourself up with meats and veggies.

Stick to the method that you are most comfortable with- as discussed; there are some ways to do intermittent fasting. Play around with all of them and get what suits you best. Make sure you try out all methods- you might be surprised which will be easiest to follow. To make something part of your lifestyle, you need to be fully comfortable with it. Intermittent fasting is no different.

Book 2: Intermittent Fasting for Women

How to Lose Weight While Traveling- Without Affecting Your Schedule

By

Beatrice Anahata

Introduction

Congratulations on grabbing your copy of *Intermittent Fasting for Women: How to Lose Weight While Traveling-Without Affecting Your Schedule* and thank you for doing so.

The following chapters will discuss what intermittent fasting is and how it works. You will learn the different methods for intermittent fasting and how you can apply them while you are traveling. Intermittent fasting can be a great help to people who are trying to lose weight while on the go.

When you are traveling, you are much less likely to eat a healthy, balanced diet. Most foods that are easily accessible while on the go are filled with processed ingredients, fat, and carbs. This is why many people gain weight while traveling. Intermittent fasting can help you balance the number of calories you are taking in each day by employing a fast then feast dietary plan.

When you are going to eat while traveling, it can be difficult to make healthy choices. Whether you are attending a banquet or eating out with friends or family, you are going to have a hard time sticking to a healthy diet. This is why several chapters of this book are dedicated to teaching you how to make healthy food choices while away from home. The book will discuss ways to eat healthier at fast food restaurants while on the road, quick snacks and meals you can have while at your hotel, and foods that you can eat on the go in between appointments or activities.

The overall goal of this book is not to put you on a diet, but rather to change the way you think about food and eating habits. Intermittent fasting is not a diet plan as much as it is a way of eating. It is a pattern that you use to consume your calories for the day. Combining intermittent fasting with healthier food choices will guarantee that you lose weight rather than gaining it while on your vacations, going to events, or traveling for work.

There are plenty of books on this subject on the market, thanks again for choosing this one! Every effort was made to ensure it is full of as much useful information as possible, please enjoy!

Chapter 1: How Intermittent Fasting Works

Intermittent fasting is a way to cut down on how many calories you take in each day or week. By eliminating several meals per week, you will net fewer calories. The fewer calories you take in, the more your body must rely on its current fat stores for energy, thus causing you to burn fat and lose weight.

While intermittent fasting is often used to jump start weight loss, it can also be used to maintain your weight after you reach your goals. This is not a diet plan to be done when you need to lose a few pounds. This is about making a lasting change to the way you approach food intake.

Health Concerns

As with any dietary plan that you implement, there are some health concerns to consider before starting intermittent fasting. You should always consider any health problems you currently have that can be affected by your food intake. If in doubt, contact your doctor to see if it is right for you.

If you have problems controlling your blood sugar, you may be required to eat several times per day for your health. Eliminating meals altogether may not be an option. However, you can eliminate full meals and eat foods high in complex carbs, such as oranges or juice, that will help you maintain your blood sugar without eating a full meal.

Some people take medications that must be taken with food. If you have a medication that you must take with food more than once per day, this can affect your ability to fast intermittently. Do some research and determine the absolute minimum number of calories that you must consume for the medication to work. In many cases, this will be about 200 calories. You can eat the minimum number of calories for your medication rather than a full meal, and still be somewhat fasting.

Methods of Intermittent Fasting

There are two main methods of intermittent fasting. In the first and most common method, you spend a set number of hours fasting and consume your calories during a short window of time each day. A common rule is 16/8: 16 hours fasting and 8 hours to eat your calories for the day. If you want to limit your calorie intake further, you might employ an 18/6 or 20/4 rule.

The other method for intermittent fasting is to fast for a full 24-hour period up to two or three times per week. For example, you might decide to eat only every other day. This method of intermittent fasting can work well if you are able to go many hours without eating. However, if you have health concerns to consider, it may not be feasible. It is much healthier overall to use the first method of intermittent fasting.

Using the 16/8 Rule

Most people who use the 16/8 rule fast from 8:00 p.m. until 12:00 p.m. the next day, creating a window for food between 12:00 p.m. and 8:00 p.m. This allows you to skip breakfast and eat lunch and dinner as well as some snacks. Some people prefer breakfast to start their day and might fast from 4:00 p.m. to 8:00 a.m., with a food window between 8:00 a.m. and 4:00 p.m., covering breakfast and lunch.

It is up to you when your food window will be. The important thing here is that you have a set time when you will eat, and a set time when you will fast. You do not want to eat breakfast, fast lunch, then eat dinner.

If you decide to go with an 18/6 or 20/4 rule, you'll use the same philosophy. With an 18/6 rule, you'll eat one meal and a snack or two each day. With the 20/4 rule, you'll eat one meal and maybe one snack each day.

You can eat at any time during your food window. It doesn't have to be a meal time. You can eat several small meals during your window, or one or two large meals. You could have a snack or two and then an average meal. It's completely up to you how you want to plan your fasting and food window.

Using the 24-Hour Fast

If you prefer not to skip meals every day, you might consider a 24-hour fast two or three times per week. For example, you would eat normally on day one, then fast from 12:00 a.m. to 12:00 a.m. on day two. Day three you would eat normally. You could then eat normally on day four and fast on day five, or fast on day four and alternate fasting and feasting days.

Again, it's up to you how you want to plan your dietary schedule and how frequently you want to fast. If you use this method, you will want to fast at least two days per week to see a benefit from it.

Occasional Fasting

Occasional fasting is the easiest kind of intermittent fasting. Basically, there is no plan, no rules. You simply skip a meal whenever it seems appropriate. If you have a huge meal for lunch, skip dinner. If you have one day where you really blow your diet and consume a ton of calories, fast until dinner the next day.

With this method, there are absolutely no rules to when and how you fast. Just keep in mind that you never want to fast for more than 24 hours straight. Fasting for longer periods can lead to health risks, including glucose depletion.

Why It Works

Your body behaves differently when it is fasting than it does when it is feasting. When you eat, your digestive system turns the food that you are eating into energy. It takes energy to digest the food as well, so depending on what you are eating, you might not get a lot of energy from the food. This is one reason why you feel tired after a big meal.

For several hours after you eat, your body continues to make use of the energy that was provided by the food. When you eat a normal three meals per day, by the time you consume your next meal, your body is just starting to get into its stores for energy. This is why it is difficult to lose weight.

When you are fasting, your body doesn't have food to use to create energy. Instead, it must turn to its own stores to create this energy. The first source that the body hits up for energy is fat stored in the cells. Therefore, you burn fat when you fast. Your body still needs energy to function, and the fat is where it gets that energy.

The body does not start to use fat stores to produce energy until four to six hours after you finish a meal. Therefore, if you are using the 16/8 method, your body will be burning fat for ten to twelve hours. If you are sleeping during those hours, your body will not burn as much fat because less energy is needed. But, if you are awake during a good portion of those hours, you can burn a lot of fat very quickly.

Intermittent fasting also teaches your body to utilize food more efficiently. It all has to do with insulin production and sensitivity. Insulin is what allows your body to transform that food into energy. When you fast, insulin production is stopped. When next you eat after a fast, your body is more sensitive to and ready for the insulin.

The end result of this process is that your body makes better use of the food you eat. Much more of the food will be converted to energy and less into fat. This way you are not only burning fat during your fasts, but you are preventing new fat to accumulate during your feasting periods.

The effects of intermittent fasting can be most fully realized when you fast through a workout session and break the fast shortly after. Your body will be prime and ready for the insulin produced by the intake of food, and the food will be much better utilized by the body.

How to Fast

Knowing how to fast seems fairly simple. After all, it just means that you don't eat, right? Actually, fasting means that you don't take in any calories during that window of time. This is easier said than done, depending on your beverage preferences.

Some free beverages that you can have without breaking your fast are diet sodas, black coffee, green tea, unsweetened black tea, and water. Any of these beverages do not have any calories, and therefore you are not breaking your fast if you have them. Diet soda is on the fence really, because while you aren't taking in any calories, you are getting quite a bit of sodium and other macros.

Now it is entirely up to you if you decide to add calorie-filled drinks to your list of acceptable beverages during your fasting periods. However, keep in mind that calories can really add up. You should definitely stay away from sweet tea and soft drinks while you are fasting, as the sugars in these beverages can add up to hundreds of calories a day very quickly.

However, if you are used to putting some creamer in your coffee, you might be okay to do that during your fasting periods. A good rule of thumb is to avoid taking in more than 100 calories during your fasting window. If you're only adding a tablespoon of flavored creamer to three or four cups of coffee in the morning, you're really not going to go over that 100 calories.

A good key to fasting is to drink plenty of water. Often, we will feel hungry when really the body just needs more hydration. Drinking a lot of water will keep you hydrated and will help stop you from breaking your fast early. It will also keep your stomach full of fluids, which will keep you from feeling hungry.

If you find that you are having a hard time with fasting and you really want to eat, you're probably focusing too much on the fact that you are fasting. Find something to do that will get your mind off of it. Read a good book, pick up a hobby like knitting or crocheting, beef up your travel itinerary to include more site seeing and window shopping trips. Do whatever you must to keep yourself busy.

Supplements are also okay while you are fasting. These do not have any calories, just nutrients that will help you throughout your day. There is absolutely nothing wrong with taking supplements and nutrients while you are fasting. The thing you are trying most to avoid is calories, fat and carbs. However, vitamins and minerals like a multi-vitamin or iron should be taken during your feasting window, because they are fat soluble and will be better utilized by your body after you have eaten.

How to Feast

During your feasting periods, you will want to keep some key points in mind. First, remember that the point of this exercise is to cut back on the number of calories that you are consuming. If you consume 2,000 calories during your feasting window, you're not going to see the benefits of intermittent fasting.

It is important that you choose healthy snacks and foods during your feasting periods. You want to feel full, but the types of foods you choose could make an enormous difference in your results. If you choose foods wisely, you'll be able to eat your fill without going overboard on calories.

The maximum number of calories that you can eat and still lose weight will depend on several factors. You'll need to take into consideration how much you weigh now and what your weight loss goals are. How many pounds do you want to lose per week?

A healthy rate of weight loss is between two and five pounds per week. Calculating based on three pounds per week, the average person should take in no more than 1,350 calories per day to lose weight. If you want to lose weight faster, you'll want to lower that amount considerably.

Keep in mind that your body does need food for energy and sustenance. If you are already fasting and then you eat less than 1,000 calories per day during your feasting window, you're going to find that you do not have the energy to do the things you need to each day.

Once you meet your weight loss goals, or if your goal is simply to maintain your weight, you can eat around 1,800 to 2,000 calories per day. The USDA recommends that you do not exceed 2,000 calories, even if you are at your goal weight. Consuming over 2,000 calories will lead to weight gain.

It is a good idea to keep track of your food intake throughout the day to make sure you don't go over on calories. It can also help you track fat and carb intake, so you can see where you might need to make healthier food choices. You can get one of any number of apps for your smart phone that will allow you to easily track your metrics.

Common Concerns

A lot of people have some concerns about fasting for any period of time. There are always questions about hunger, fatigue, and possible negative effects. Here are some quick answers to put your mind at ease.

You will feel very hungry while you are fasting—at first. Your body has been trained to eat every so often, and therefore your brain will tell you it is time to eat. After the first week or so of intermittent fasting, this immense hunger will go away. Your body will get used to getting food only a couple of times a day, and it will adjust accordingly.

As for fatigue, you really won't feel any difference in energy levels by fasting. Your body will find the energy it needs to function. This is why intermittent fasting works. Your body creates energy from fat stores when no food is consumed. Energy is necessary to life, and the body will find a way to create what is needed.

Another concern that people have is that their body will go into starvation mode and begin to store extra calories instead of burning them. This is simply not going to happen with intermittent fasting. While it is true that your body can go into starvation mode after prolonged fasting and cause you to gain fat stores, this does not happen with short fasts such as intermittent fasting. With between a sixteen and 24-hour fast, your body will not go into starvation mode.

Chapter 2: Deciding When to Fast While Traveling

After the first chapter, you should have a basic idea of how you want to do your intermittent fasting on a regular basis. Unfortunately, when you're traveling, you aren't always able to keep up your normal eating habits. It can be quite a chore to stick to a dietary plan or schedule while on the go.

The key here is to be prepared. Consider the challenges you will face sticking to your intermittent fasting schedule and diet while you are traveling. When you know what you're dealing with, you can plan around it. It is perfectly okay to change your fasting and feasting schedule to meet the needs of your busy life.

If you are planning on trying intermittent fasting for the first time while traveling, keep in mind that you will feel hungry during your fast for the first few days. Try to keep your fasting times to times that you will be in a plane or car, or times when you will be extremely busy so that you can't think about the fact that you aren't eating.

Itinerary

Take a close look at your itinerary. During what time of day will you be on the road most of the time? What events do you have planned that are going to include food? All these things are going to need to be considered carefully to determine when you should fast while on your vacation or business trip.

If you're going to primarily be on the road during the morning and early afternoon, you might consider that your fasting period include those hours. It is extremely difficult to make healthy food choices while on the road. Convenience food is often processed and filled with unhealthy carbs and fats and tends to be higher in calories.

If you are attending events that will include food, make sure that your feasting period covers those times. For example, you don't want your fasting period to be from 8:00 p.m. to 12:00 p.m. if you know you are going to be attending a brunch at 11:00 a.m. You may have to adjust your normal feasting and fasting periods to account for these events.

On the other hand, don't be overly concerned if you must break your fast a little bit early. Breaking your fast a half hour to an hour early isn't going to have a detrimental effect on the benefits of intermittent fasting. If it is too difficult to adjust your eating schedule, or it's just for one day, it really isn't a big deal to break fast a tad bit earlier than originally planned.

It is important that you plan your fasting around the events that will have food. Especially if you're just starting out with intermittent fasting, being around food during your fasting period will be excruciatingly difficult. Rather than torture yourself and risk ruining your dietary streak, plan ahead to be feasting during these times.

If you will be attending events throughout the day that include food, you may have to dismiss complete fasting. However, you can still limit your calorie intake. If your itinerary has you having breakfast at 9:00 a.m., luncheon at 12:00 p.m., and a dinner banquet at 6:00 p.m., you might find it difficult to fast completely.

Instead of torturing yourself with being around food while fasting, consider grazing. If you would normally be fasting during breakfast, try to have just coffee and maybe a single egg or some fruit. If you are eating something light without a lot of calories, it is going to still net you fewer calories than if you weren't fasting at all. This way you can be eating with your guests or hosts, but not completely sabotage your efforts.

Another good idea is to plan your itinerary around your fasting periods as much as possible. For example, if your colleagues are going to be having brunch before a seminar, skip the brunch and do some site seeing, arriving back at the conference center in time for the seminar. This way you can fast comfortably without affecting your overall schedule.

Workouts

Remember that you want to break your fast soon after a workout. Sometimes when you're traveling, it can be difficult if not impossible to get an actual workout in. But you can still use this philosophy to a point.

Are you going site seeing? Are you going to be walking around an amusement park? Will you be shopping? Any of these things can be considered exercise. If these are part of your itinerary, you should plan to break you fast soon after you stop the exercise for the day, or after a lengthy session.

If you're going to an amusement park, this might mean fasting throughout the day, and breaking fast around 4:00 p.m. when you stop for the night. It really depends on how much you will be moving and at what point during the day the movement will be slowing down. Remember that this is entirely up to you when you fast and when you break that fast.

If you're spending a large portion of your traveling on the road or in a plane, you're not going to get much exercise in. When that happens, base your fasting and feasting periods on other factors. It's okay to miss a workout a few days while you are traveling.

Available Foods

It can take some digging for this next step of preparation for your vacation or business trip. When you are traveling, you are often at the mercy of your hosts, the hotel, and the local restaurants as to what exactly you will be eating. What you will be eating

115

should play a role in determining when and how long to fast while traveling.

Remember that one of the primary goals of intermittent fasting is to take in fewer calories within each 24-hour period. If you are going to be consuming many calories in a short period of time, you may need to fast for a longer period prior to the feast. This way you will still net fewer calories but will be able to enjoy your vacation experience.

Research

You'll want to start by getting the menu for the hotel you will be staying in. What healthy food choices are available in the dining room or room service? If everything on the menu appears to be high in fat, carbs, and calories, you might want to consider planning ahead and avoiding the hotel food. However, most hotels today recognize that people have dietary concerns and have healthier food choices available.

It is also a good idea to take a look at what restaurants are in the area you will be traveling to, and plan in advance which ones you will go to. Check out what their menus are online and choose the best restaurants with the healthiest food. Sometimes your itinerary will not allow you the luxury of stopping at a particular restaurant, so make sure you take that into account.

You should also get the menus for any brunches, luncheons, or dinner banquets you will be attending while traveling. You have little or no choice about what you eat at these events but knowing ahead of time what will be available could make a difference in when and how long you fast while you are traveling.

If you will be staying with a host, or going to a private dinner party, relay your dietary needs to the host. While they may not be able to accommodate you fully, they should be able to make some allowances to keep foods from being too full of calories, such as leaving off sauces from your meal.

You'll also want to take into consideration what they are serving, and how much you will eat of it.

Don't forget when doing this research and planning, to also consider the snacks and desserts that are going to be offered to you. While you certainly don't need to eat everything you are offered, it can be impolite to turn down something such as wedding cake, birthday cake, or an award-winning pie.

Planning

Once you have a solid idea of what foods will be available to you, you can work on planning when and how long you will fast while traveling. You will want to carefully consider the quality and calorie content of the food that you will be eating.

For example, if you are going to a wedding and there will be a banquet after, you should have gotten the menu for the banquet. Let's say that the menu includes only high calorie, high fat foods that are going to really add up fast. You don't want to limit yourself at the banquet and be hungry later while you should be fasting, but you also don't want to consume too many calories during your feasting period.

In this case, you would want to plan on fasting for a longer period of time on that particular day. If you know you are going to consume your 1,300 calories at that one event, fast from after dinner the night before until the event itself. This way you are still netting fewer calories overall and you will not be sabotaging your weight loss goals.

To help you control your appetite and food intake during those meals that are high in calories, you can make use of the rest of your feasting period for the day to eat small, healthy snacks. Have some fruit to break your fast, and snack on fruit or crackers throughout the period. Maybe you could have a protein bar as well, a couple of hours before the larger meal. This will keep you from feeling too hungry and consuming too many calories during the big feast.

Sticking to the Plan

When you put so much time and effort into making a plan for your fasting and feasting, it is that much easier to stick to it when the time comes. After all, if you don't stick to your plan, that's a lot of wasted time and effort. However, plans can change, and you must be ready and willing to roll with the punches.

For example, you might get to the conference center on a business trip and discover that the itinerary has completely changed from what you were told in advance. They may now be offering food during your fasting periods. Use your willpower to avoid breaking your fast too early. Find other activities to do away from the offered food if possible, or simply politely turn it down.

You might get to a restaurant and find that the menu you found online isn't accurate, and you aren't able to stick to your calorie restrictions. When this happens, you might not have the time to find another restaurant with a healthier menu. Instead, go ahead and get the healthiest item possible that you will enjoy. If you go significantly over your planned calorie intake, simply start your fast immediately after the meal instead of a couple of hours later. For instance, if you are feasting from 12:00 p.m. to 8:00 p.m. and you're having the dinner at 6:00 p.m., start your fast at 7:00 p.m. instead of 8:00 p.m. You might add an hour or two to the other end of your fast as well.

Be prepared for things to change, but to stick to your overall plan regardless of the changes in your schedule and menu. This will help you be more successful with your intermittent fasting so that you can continue to work on your weight loss goals while traveling.

Chapter 3: Fast Food on the Road

One of the biggest pitfalls to trying to lose weight while traveling is the quality of food available to you while on the road. Long road trips by necessity require convenience or fast food, especially if you are on a tight schedule. Most of the places you'll be able to get food during your feasting periods while on the road are not going to be of the best quality.

There are, however, some easy ways that you can eat this fast food and convenience food and not gain weight. You just have to make healthier choices. It can be difficult if you are stopping at fast food restaurants, but it can be done with careful determination.

Fast Food

The biggest problems with fast food are sauces, breads, potatoes, and fried foods. If you can avoid these, you will still be able to lose weight while traveling. You may be thinking, "What else is there to eat at a fast food restaurant?" The answer is, you have to make your own menu by asking for special order meals.

Many fast food restaurants today offer side salads on their menu. These aren't the best quality salads, but they are edible, and they are a nice small side item. If you aren't the one driving, or if you have time to stop and eat inside the restaurant, substituting a salad for fries or onion rings can go a long way toward helping keep you under your calorie requirements. Just remember that salad dressing adds a ton of calories, so always ask for whatever light dressing they have.

Burger Joints

As for the main dish, avoid sandwiches of any kind. You might think that you are doing good to order a grilled chicken sandwich because it isn't fried and doesn't have breading. However, by the time you add the bun and the sauces, you've got quite a lot of calories.

Most fast food restaurants only offer sandwiches. So, what are you to do? Order the sandwich without the bread or sauce. Essentially, you are getting just a piece of grilled chicken with a slice of tomato and some lettuce. The cashier might give you a funny look, but they will fulfill your request. You can do the same thing with hamburgers. However, you should not get any fried chicken or fish.

If you are worried about being able to eat your bun-less food in the car, make sure you get the piece of grilled chicken and pat it dry with napkins before leaving drive thru. This will make the chicken dry enough that you won't get your fingers messy just picking it up and eating it like you would a sandwich.

Taco Places

If you stop at a fast food restaurant such as a Taco Bell or other Mexican place, you'll need to take a slightly different approach. It is a good idea to stick to tacos when you go to a restaurant like this. Tacos are basically just seasoned meat, cheese, lettuce, maybe tomato, and a tortilla shell. It is the lowest calorie item on the menu in most cases.

Avoid burritos and specialty items. These items typically have more carbs from both a larger tortilla or multiple layers of tortilla, as well as from sauces. Avoid cheese sauces, as these are very high in calories and fat.

Seafood Places

It is best to avoid seafood fast food places as much as possible. You're going to find it very difficult to find anything on the menu that isn't fried. You're definitely not going to find anything that's not fried that can be eaten in the car.

If you absolutely must eat at a seafood place, do it only if you have the time to sit inside and eat rather than on the go. Most of these places do have a baked fish option that might come with rice or veggies. Just make sure that you skip the hush puppies, fries, and fried okra.

Truck Stops and Diners

There is a reason these are called grease pits! Everything you get from most truck stops and diners is covered in grease. Avoid these restaurants if you can, but if you get outvoted or it's the only thing around, you do have some options.

Again, you want to avoid breads and fried foods as much as possible. Don't get the greasy hamburger and fries! You'll want to focus instead on other menu options. Some diners and truck stops have a partial menu on the table, and you have to ask to get a full menu. If you don't see a healthy option on the menu you are given or that is at the table, ask the waitress if there is another menu available.

Luckily, most truck stops and diners offer breakfast all day. This is good news because breakfast food is going to have the least amount of fat and carbs if you're careful. Always order eggs and ask that they be cooked with light oil or grease. You don't have to limit yourself to egg whites unless you are really counting your calories for that meal.

To go along with your eggs, see if they have an option to substitute fruit for the hash browns that almost always come with eggs at these restaurants. If they don't have a fruit option, skip the side altogether. You might get yourself a side of sausage patties, as these can easily be patted dry of excess grease and has less fat than bacon. Avoid toast, biscuits, and gravy.

Some diners and truck stops might also offer baked or grilled chicken or baked or grilled fish. If this is an option for you, make sure that you don't get any sauces on your meat, and choose only vegetables for the sides. Avoid potatoes that are filled with starch and loaded with calorie-filled toppings.

Another option is to get the burger, but without the bun and toppings. If you go this route, you'll want to ask for extra napkins. Pat the burger dry of all grease to cut down on the amount of fat that you are consuming. Make sure you get veggies as a side and not fries or other potatoes.

One thing that a lot of truck stops and small diners are known for is pie. You will undoubtedly be asked if you'd like dessert or a slice of pie. Just say no! If you really feel that you absolutely must have a bite of pie, see if you can split a piece with the person you are traveling with.

Convenience Foods

There may be times during your travels when there aren't any restaurants around when you need to eat, and you wind up stopping at a convenience store. Convenience food is the worst for your diet and health. Chips, donuts, candy, and roller grill items are filled with carbs and fat.

There usually are some healthier choices at convenience stores if you're willing to pay for them. Unfortunately, the healthier foods at these stores are almost always more expensive than the junk food. But, sticking to your diet and furthering your weight loss goals is worth it, right?

Look first to see if they have protein bars. Protein bars are often lower in carbs than much of the other foods that will be available at these stores. They also have a high amount of protein and a few healthy fats, which will go a long way toward filling you up more, so that you eat less.

Another good go-to is fruit. Not all convenience stores have fruit, but most of them will at least have bananas. Grab a banana or two, or an apple to tide you over to your next available stop with a real meal.

Another good convenience store food that you can try is hot dogs or sausages without the bun. The bun and toppings are really what is going to get you on these roller grill items. Some convenience stores have other items available as well, such as cheeseburger rolls or buffalo chicken rolls, which are even healthier for you—again, without the bun and toppings.

Trail mix is another great go-to food that you'll always be able to find in convenience stores. Just take note of what is in the trail mix and look at the nutritional facts before choosing one. Some trail mix has a lot of candy mixed in or is made with artificial ingredients. Trail mix of dried fruit, raisins, nuts, and sunflower seeds are really the best. A good trail mix is low calorie, low fat, low carb, and filling.

While you're at the convenience store make sure you stock up on water, vitamin water, juice, and maybe milk. Beverages will keep you hydrated, and juice and milk will give you additional vitamins and nutrients that will help keep you going until you can eat a real meal at another stop.

Make sure that you are avoiding the really carb filled and sugar filled items like candy bars, chips, and soft drinks. Diet drinks are okay if you really need something with caffeine to stay awake on the road, but black coffee is much better for you. If you really want something a bit salty for a snack, look to see if they have some kind of low carb snack cracker, like Wheat Thins.

Chapter 4: Dining Out and Event Banquets

There will be times when you are traveling that you may not have much control over where you take in your meals. When you are at the mercy of the decisions of others, it can be difficult to make healthy eating choices that support your weight loss. When you don't get to pick the restaurant, or you are attending a banquet, you'll have to be a little more creative about watching what you eat.

Banquets are a bit easier to deal with than dining out at restaurants because you will often be given a choice in what you want to eat at a banquet in advance. If you're able to RSVP with your dinner choice, make sure you choose the option that is the healthiest, with the lowest calories, carbs, and fat. If the banquet is served buffet style this is even better because you will have complete control over what you put on your plate.

When eating at restaurants, don't be afraid to order your meal with special instructions. Do not feel obligated to take the meal exactly as it is typically prepared. If everything on the menu is covered in fatty sauces, request your meal sans sauce. If something comes with a potato, ask to substitute for vegetables or fruit. Most restaurants are extremely accommodating.

Portion Sizes

One of the best things you can do to watch your weight while traveling is monitor your portion sizes. Americans have the largest portion sizes of any country when it comes to restaurants and banquets. Nowhere else in the world serves as much food at one time as Americans do. This is one reason why obesity is so prevalent in America.

We were always told as children to eat everything on our plates. This rule has been so ingrained in us that we tend to eat whatever amount we have been given, or until we are so full we simply cannot take another bite. You must break this habit when eating at restaurants and banquets, or you will not be able to stick to your calorie restrictions.

You must convince yourself that it is perfectly okay to leave food behind. Do not feel like you must finish your entire meal to be polite. Especially for carb rich or high calorie meals, it is important that you only eat the portion of the food in front of you that meets your calorie intake goals. It is perfectly okay to leave the rest behind.

As a rule, you will want to eat about half of the food that you are given at a restaurant or banquet unless the portion sizes are very reasonable. This is particularly true of Italian restaurants and steak houses. The amount of food that you are given at these restaurants is often twice what you should be eating.

One option that you might have depending on the restaurant, is to order from the kids or seniors menu. These menus often have smaller portion sizes. Most restaurants offer the same meals on the senior menu as the regular menu, just in smaller sizes. While the restaurant may not allow you to pay the senior price if you are not of the right age, you can often offer to pay full price, but request the senior portion sizes.

If you are being served at a banquet and it is being served buffet style, don't be afraid to speak up and tell the servers exactly what you want. Ask for the smallest piece of meat. Ask for an extra spoonful of veggies. Request that they cut a large potato in half. The servers are there to help you, and there is nothing wrong with making sure you get the portions that you will be able to eat on your diet.

A typical meal should consist of three to four ounces of meat, one cup of vegetables, and one small starch such as a dinner roll or small potato. For things like pasta, a portion should consist of about a cup. It can be difficult to eyeball these measurements without practice but keeping this in mind will go a long way toward helping you maintain control of your diet.

Foods to Avoid

There are some foods that you will want to avoid as much as possible when eating at a restaurant or banquet. These foods are high in fat and add tons of unnecessary calories to your meal. When possible, ask for your meal to exclude these items.

Sauces

The healthiest foods can be made unhealthy simply by adding sauces and other toppings. Cheese sauces are very high in fat and can add 100 calories or more to your meal. Gravies and butter rich sauces are also culprits to watch for.

If you are dining in a restaurant, ask for your meat, veggies, and potatoes to be served without sauce or gravy. Avoid dishes that cannot be easily prepared by altering the recipe to omit the sauce. This includes things like pasta.

If you are eating at a banquet, the sauce may already be on the food that you are getting, and you may not be able to get it without. When this happens, accept a smaller portion of the food. If you can, such as with meats, scrape off the sauce after you sit down with your plate.

Potatoes

Americans love meat and potatoes meals. Potatoes are a high starch food and contain almost nothing but carbs. They have very little nutritional value, especially if you are not eating the skin.

What really makes potatoes bad for you at a restaurant or banquet is that they are almost never served just as a plain old potato. Baked potatoes might be loaded with chives, butter, and sour cream, making them even higher in calories and unhealthier. Mashed potatoes are often loaded with milk or cream, lots of butter, and potentially gravy.

Other potato dishes are covered in cheese, such as scalloped potatoes. All of these variations of potato are high in calories and fat and should be left off of your plate whenever possible. If you have limited food choices and feel compelled to take a serving of potatoes at a banquet, make sure that you only accept a half portion, or eat only half of what you are served.

Vegetables

Why would you want to avoid vegetables? They are supposed to be healthy, right? The problem is that often at banquets vegetables are cooked with an insane amount of butter. This adds a lot of unwanted calories and fat to your meal. Creamed vegetables made with the whole cream are also very bad for you and will work against your weight loss goals.

Whenever possible at a restaurant, request steamed vegetables that are not cooked with any butter or added fats. When this is not possible, or if the vegetables are being served at a banquet where no steamed option is available, consider going without the veggies or get a smaller portion size.

All restaurants and most banquets will offer salad. This is a much healthier choice if the vegetables are made with a lot of fat. However, keep in mind that your salad can also be unhealthy if you cover it in cheese, bacon pieces, meats, and dressings. Choose vinegar and oil or a light Italian dressing over fatty dressings like ranch or blue cheese.

Pastas

Pasta is a carb rich food with little nutritional value on its own, but what really makes pasta bad for you is the sauces that are added to it. Avoid things like macaroni and cheese or other pasta bakes at banquets.

If you find yourself in an Italian restaurant, consider ordering soup rather than pasta dishes. Some Italian restaurants also have a steak option, but again, you need to be careful of what sides you order with it. If you decide to go with soup, look carefully at the descriptions of the soups available and choose one that does not use heavy cream or other fats.

Breads

Nearly every meal you are served in a restaurant will come with some form of bread. Some restaurants serve a loaf of bread family style, others provide a basket full of unlimited dinner rolls or breadsticks, and others serve the meal with a dinner roll. Everywhere you look at a restaurant or banquet there will be bread of some kind.

Bread is very high in carbs and provides little nutritional value unless it is whole grain. A lot of breads served by fancier restaurants and banquets are made with whole cream or other fats, honey, and other sugars. The cooks then load the bread down with butter or honey on top and serve it with yet more butter.

Whenever you are at a restaurant, turn down the bread. Tell the server to omit the bread from your meal or ignore the pile of bread on the table. At banquets, you can simply ignore the bread or refuse it at the buffet line.

Desserts

When others at your table in a restaurant are getting dessert, it can be very tempting to get some yourself. Desserts in restaurants are usually very rich and can consist of as many calories as the meal itself in some cases. It is best to skip the dessert altogether most of the time.

Some restaurants offer sugar free desserts, and these can often be much better for you. Be careful though that you don't choose a sugar free dessert made with heavy cream because this will also have a lot of calories. Sugar free fruit pie is a good choice if you must have dessert.

When at a banquet such as for a wedding or other celebration, there will undoubtedly be cake, and everyone is expected to have a piece. If you feel you must out of politeness, go ahead and have a small piece of cake. Have the piece cut small, then scrape off the excess frosting or icing and candies that decorate it.

Chapter 5: Quick Meals and Snacks for the Hotel

While some hotels offer meal services, they are often costly and limited in options. When you are staying at a hotel that does not offer meal services, or the options are not healthy, you might have to plan some quick meals and snacks that you can have at the beginning or end of your feasting period.

The meal and snack choices listed in this chapter are easily found at the local grocery store, even if you are in a small town or tourist town. Depending on the time of year, you might even be able to get some foods at a local farmers market and make it part of your site seeing and shopping experience.

If you know that you are going to take this option for food while traveling, plan ahead by looking up where the local grocery stores are in relation to your hotel so that you can save time when you are actually in the city you are traveling to. This way you're not spending unnecessary time searching for what you need when you get there.

If the hotel does offer meal services and has some options, choose carefully to make sure you stick to your dietary and calorie restrictions. Hotels are often not as eager to make changes to the meals, so special ordering something may be out of the question. There are still some healthy options however, depending on the offerings of the hotel kitchen.

Do It Yourself Meals and Snacks

When a hotel offers a mini fridge or microwave in the room, it makes things much easier in this respect. While not all hotels offer a mini fridge, most hotels today do offer a microwave in the room. If a microwave is not available in the room itself, there may be one available in the lounge or dining area.

If there is not a mini fridge in the room, your options for quick meals and snacks will be more limited. However, you can also plan ahead by bringing along a cooler to keep some small items in for later use. There are also insulated tote bags that work well for this. When using these items, it is best to get freezer cold packs rather than actual ice to reduce mess as it melts. They also last longer than bagged ice in most cases.

Fruits and Vegetables

There are a lot of fruits and vegetables that do not have to be kept refrigerated. Apples, oranges, and bananas are good choices to take with you, or purchase to eat at the hotel for breakfasts or a light lunch or snack. If you have a mini fridge or cooler tote, you can also make use of things like grapes, berries, and melons.

Many vegetables also don't have to be refrigerated. Hotels are often kept cool enough that things like carrots, broccoli, and cauliflower will not go bad for up to 24 hours if they are kept in a cool dry place. They do not necessarily have to be kept refrigerated.

If you want to spruce up your veggies, try getting a veggie dip. Avoid ranch as it is high in calories. However, a good avocado dip or hummus is good with vegetables and keeps fairly well in a mini fridge or insulated tote bag.

Cheese and Crackers

Cheese and crackers is a good light lunch to break your fast if you start your feasting period in the morning, or before you are leaving the hotel. Cheese can be kept in a mini fridge or cooler tote. Some cheeses are okay to leave unrefrigerated as long as they don't get warm, but this is not ideal.

Since you are in a hotel and won't have use of a kitchen and utensils, it is a good idea to buy small cheese trays rather than a block of cheese. The cheese trays are often available in a small one-pound variety pack, already sliced perfectly for use with crackers. Other options are cheese sticks and cheese slices.

Peanut Butter and Jelly

Peanut butter and jelly made with low carb bread or flat bread is a good choice for a light lunch or snack before bed. Peanut butter and most jellies do not have to be kept refrigerated, and it is very easy to prepare. You can also use peanut butter on your apples or some celery, which also do not have to be kept very cold.

Instant Meals

There are a lot of nutritious instant foods out there that do not require refrigeration but can be prepared with hot water from the coffee pot in your room, or with a microwave. Instant oatmeal is a great way to break your fast in the morning or early afternoon and doesn't require much in the way of preparation.

There are also a variety of soups that are designed to be cooked in the microwave. Campbell's makes an excellent line of microwaveable soup cups that are delicious and nutritious. These can make an excellent light supper, or snack at the end of your feasting period at the end of your long day.

Deli Meats

If you have a mini fridge in your room or are making use of an insulated tote, you can get some deli meats to have for a lunch or dinner in your hotel room. You can roll up the meat with some lettuce and tomato for a low carb meal, or you can use low carb bread or tortillas to make a sandwich or wrap.

Keep in mind when making deli sandwiches that it is only as healthy as what you put on it. Using a lot of mayonnaise or whipped salad dressing could add calories that you don't want to worry about counting. Be careful too, what breads you choose for sandwiches, as many breads served in delis are high in carbs and fat.

Eating at the Hotel Kitchen

Eating in the dining room or with room service at the hotel is always an option. If you have a very busy itinerary, and don't have a chance to eat your main meal until you return to the hotel for the night, the hotel kitchen can be a good choice. Just check ahead and make sure what hours the kitchen is open and room service is available.

Luckily, hotel dining is usually smaller portion sizes than your typical restaurant, so you won't have to worry about eating too much when you order from the hotel kitchen. Still, you will have to make sure that you are making healthy food choices. This can be easier said than done because often hotels will not make alterations to the presentation of the food. You must order it the way it comes, or not at all.

The trick here is to choose items that are not going to be high in fat or carbs. Avoid fried foods and potatoes, above all. You should also be careful that when ordering meat dishes, they do not come with sauces made with heavy creams or other fats.

One of the easiest to order and healthiest meals you can get from a hotel kitchen is a steak dinner. Their steaks are usually smaller than at a steak house, so you won't risk overeating. They often come with steamed vegetables and a potato, but you can always simply not eat the potato. Another good option is baked or grilled chicken with vegetables.

One way that you might be able to save yourself some calories when eating at the hotel kitchen is to order breakfast fare. Frequently, hotels will serve their full menu all day, catering to those on a different schedule than the average person. If breakfast is an option at any time of day, you're in luck. A good meal is an order of eggs with sausage and a side of fruit, with perhaps an English muffin.

Another good option for hotel kitchens is a salad. They often have a variety of salads to choose from, including tuna and egg salad. If you are eating it as a heavy meal for lunch or dinner, you can get a chef salad with ham and hard-boiled eggs, or you could get a grilled chicken salad. Always keep in mind that the dressing is what kills you on a salad and ask for the lightest option available.

Of course, if you've been good about sticking to your fasting schedule and you haven't consumed too many calories, the smaller portion sizes of hotel kitchens make it so that you can splurge a bit on a late dinner. If nutrition facts aren't listed on the menu, try using a calorie counter app on your smart phone or tablet to determine how many calories are in the meal you really want. It's perfectly okay to splurge a bit in the evening if you've been really good about your calorie intake all day.

Chapter 6: Quick Snacks on the Go

If you are traveling long distances on a flight or in a car, it can be helpful to snack your way through your feasting periods. This way you are not having to worry about the high calorie options at fast food restaurants, diners, and convenience stores along the way.

Snacking your way through your feasting period is also a good option if you are in a city while you are traveling and have a tight schedule. If you are trying to cram as much as possible into a short vacation, or if you are on a business trip with a lot of meetings, quick snacks are a great way to get in your calories for the day. You can snack while on the bus, in the taxi, on the train, or in between meetings.

The following snacks are ones that are very healthy and won't add up too quickly on the calorie front. They are easy to transport and do not require refrigeration at all. If you know you are going to be very busy or on a long trip, you might consider packing a tote with some or all of these foods to tide you over during your travels.

Food for Energy

Complex carbs are a great source of energy and can keep you alert on long car rides. These quick snacks are a great alternative to simple carbs and sugars but will give you the energy you need to stay focused and navigate your way to your destination. Or, they will give you energy for site seeing, shopping, and other activities.

Fresh fruit is always a good choice for complex carbs. There is a lot of fruit that you can get that doesn't have to be refrigerated, including apples, oranges, and bananas. If you're packing a heavy tote, apples can be best because they won't get crushed by other items in your bag or car.

If you prefer something that you don't have to worry about going bad or getting warm, you can go with some dried fruit. Get bags of dried fruit from your local health foods store or make your own in advance of your trip. Dried cranberries, blueberries, apricots, and dates are a great super food that will keep you energized and on the go.

Trail mix is another great option. You can get trail mix with dried fruit, nuts, seeds, and raisins. Trail mix is a good choice because it provides you with complex carbs as well as protein.

Apple sauce cups are another good source of complex carbohydrates and are fairly easy to eat on the go. Just make sure you remember to pack some plastic spoons for use with anything like this that you decide to take on your travels.

Food for Protein

Proteins are important because they give you energy in much the same way as complex carbohydrates, but proteins will also make you feel fuller. Proteins are a great way to make sure that you are getting enough calories and good fats as well, since most sources of protein are also sources of these nutrients.

Jerky is the absolute best source of protein that you can take with you on your travels. It keeps well in any climate, can easily be resealed in a Ziploc bag, and can be slipped out and munched down in a matter of minutes. Jerky also comes in so many different flavors, shapes, and sizes that you'll never get bored of eating it.

Another good source of protein are protein bars. Protein bars are different than basic granola bars. Protein bars are usually made up of a whey protein powder as a part of their base and contain nuts and peanut butter most frequently. Some also contain dried fruit. These protein bars are extremely filling and give you lasting energy.

Nuts and seeds are another good source of protein and good fats, and they are a great snack food. Sometimes when you're on the road for a long time or in a flight, you get bored and want to eat. Nuts and seeds are great for this because you have to eat an awful lot of them before the calories start stacking up. And the protein will give you a full feeling faster than with sugary or carb filled snacks like chips.

Protein shakes are another great way to get your protein in and can also get you some calcium and iron as well. You can get protein shakes that do not have to be refrigerated and are pre-made. You can also get protein powder and simply add water or milk when you get to a stand or store that sells such items. A protein shake is a good option if you are going somewhere that beverages are allowed but food is not.

Cheese sticks are another source of protein and calcium that will help keep you going throughout your busy day. Most cheese sticks are okay to be out of refrigeration for a few hours before they must be eaten safely, so long as the climate is not overly warm. For example, if you have cheese sticks in your tote, you should not leave it by a heat vent.

Snack Foods

If you really just want something that's a basic light snack, are craving something a bit salty, or just want to splurge a bit, there are some snack foods that are good for on the go that aren't a lot of calories. It is best to avoid chips as much as possible, but you do have some other alternatives.

Popcorn is a great alternative to snack chips and crackers. Popcorn, even with butter, is a very low-calorie snack that you can enjoy while on the go. Put it in a Ziploc bag so that you can enjoy it throughout the day and munch whenever you have time. Popcorn isn't really going to fill you up or give you energy, but it will give you something to eat if you're really feeling like you have to have something right now.

Pretzels are another good snack alternative to chips that are fairly low in calories. Snack pretzels are a great option if you want something really salty but are trying to count your calories and carbs. You can also get snack pretzel bites that have peanut butter in them for a combination of a snack treat and protein.

When you're really feeling hungry and it's not time to eat a full meal, or if you're close to your calorie limits for the day, rice cakes can be a great light snack. Rice cakes come in a variety of flavors and don't have to taste like Styrofoam. They are somewhat filling due to the puffed-up rice, which expands further in your stomach. Rice cakes are a good way to avoid calories while still not depriving yourself of food when you want it.

Sandwiches

If you are looking for more of a meal on the go than a quick snack, a sandwich is a good option. You can easily travel with a sandwich for long periods. Deli meat sandwiches are good outside of refrigeration for up to four hours, while peanut butter and jelly sandwiches are good for a longer period of time.

Remember that when you are making your deli meat sandwiches for the road that you do not want to put any tomato on the sandwich, as this will rot over time if not eating within the first hour of taking the sandwich out of refrigeration. You also do not want to put any salad dressing, mayo, or mustard on the sandwich until you are ready to eat it or the bread will become soggy. Adding cheese to your sandwich is okay, as long as the sandwich will not be in the heat.

Peanut butter crackers are going to be a slightly higher calorie snack food, but they are a good choice if you want to combine salty with protein. Avoid processed foods and instead make your own peanut butter crackers using saltines and no sugar added peanut butter. Zip them up in a baggie and you're ready for a long trip. This is a much better choice than peanut butter and jelly sandwiches, because jelly can make the bread soggy over the course of several hours.

Avoid egg salad sandwiches because eggs go bad very quickly once taken out of refrigeration. However, tuna salad, if it does not contain eggs, can be kept unrefrigerated for several hours. However, the mayo in the tuna salad can cause bread to become soggy. Make sure you make the sandwich out of a stiff whole grain bread or carry the salad separately from the bread and bring along a plastic spoon to spread it with.

Book 3: Intermittent Fasting for Women

Trim That Belly Fat and Have Limitless Energy While Being a Full-Time Mom

By

Beatrice Anahata

Introduction

Congratulations on grabbing your copy of this book and thank you for doing so.

This book will discuss how you can incorporate Intermittent Fasting into your lifestyle. It will tell you the advantages of doing so and also the correct plans. This book is focused towards the intermittent fasting plans for full-time moms. It will widen your perspective about intermittent fasting and the positive changes it can in your life.

Being a Full-time mom is a demanding job. It is a crown of thrones. Too many expectations, demands, and too little time. From sunshine to sundown, an unending race ensues. The race to fulfill the responsibilities requires complete and undivided attention. Then, there are the blues of unfulfilled expectations. Responsibilities that went off the chart. Guilt pangs of not being able to do everything. Resentment of not being able to keep everyone happy. The frustration of family members not fully understanding or cooperating with you.

In the middle of all this, your own health keeps getting ignored. The easiest thing to sacrifice in the midst of all this is the personal time. Slowly and gradually, it does take a toll on you. That daily small amount of aerobics, yoga, meditation or walk can keep you rejuvenated. But, you don't find time for it all the time. You compromise on that time. You feel low and compensate it with food. This begins a vicious cycle. Fat accumulation accelerates. This is the beginning of the downward spiral. Once this starts, going back gets tough.

Great transformation stories, motivations speeches, Ted-talks all look good and inspiring. But, there is little time, energy and motivation to bring them into action. If you let the time pass by like this, then soon oodles of fat would accumulate. Those who think that they'll cross the bridge when they reach it are wrong. Once you cross the threshold going back is tough. Strict exercise regimen requires time. You never had it in the first place. The strict diet requires time; it was never your luxury. From weight training to healthy living, everything would start getting off limits. You will slowly and gradually compromise with the weight. It would trigger the next set of problems in form of obesity-related diseases.

All this while, there is one aspect that always bothered you but kept getting ignored. It is the negative impact of belly fat on your appearance. Being a full-time mom doesn't mean that you are any less of a woman. It makes you more of that. It is your right to look beautiful and attractive. The tire belly is not only a cosmetic problem but also a health hazard. You start feeling tired more often. Lose stamina and libido. Feel more stressed and fatigued.

You are aware of it all the time. You press the panic button in desperation. As they say, desperate times call for desperate measures. You look up the internet; talk to your friends and consult the experts. You get sound advises on reducing the belly fat and bringing your weight under control. You resolve to be firm and stick to the schedule. The workouts are tough and the family still demanding. The pressure becomes unbearable. Kids have school. Home needs care. The family needs time. You need relaxation, and the current regimen doesn't properly fit in the picture. You start making compromises, and the resolution goes out of the window.

This is the story in general of all the full-time moms who is struggling with their weight. Most succumb to pressure and make compromises. It is acceding defeat, but most had no option. Let's get real here for a moment. Being a full-time mom is a full-time responsibility. The burden is immense. The expectations are high. It isn't a walk in the garden even for the most well-off. It requires dedication, time, and determination. It asks you to sacrifice some things and ignore many. Being a responsible mom, both are difficult things.

You can lose some weight with a strict exercise regimen and strict control on your diet. But, both demand time and energy, two things on which you are already running short. Anytime you start getting lax on them you'll gain weight much faster than you lost. These are not practical ways for full-time moms who have the family as their first priority. This isn't a sustainable model. Sustainability is the name of the game when it comes to the schedule of a full-time mom. You will not remain motivated forever. A child or family member falls sick, family engagements and other things that require your attention will shift your focus. Your life will become a roller coaster ride of guilt pangs, failures, and disappointments. You need a method that makes it easier for you to control your weight. A method that doesn't require you to go off the track. That doesn't require extraordinary effort. A method that doesn't disrupt your normal course of life.

Intermittent fasting is that way that opens the doors of opportunities for it. It is easy, sustainable, and effective. Every additional activity you do like exercise, yoga, aerobics, and jogging will boost your efforts. Yet, if you are not able to devote time to them, you will still be on track. You will not have to take out extra time for preparing lengthy meals and diet plans. Your current diet will also do. Choosing to adopt a healthy diet will surely complement your weight loss efforts. It is the sustainable model for full-time moms as they can be their usual self while bringing the change.

Intermittent fasting is no magic trick. But, it is bringing harmony inside your body. It gives your body to realize its full potential. It triggers the right hormones that help in losing weight. It makes your life more disciplined and orderly.

The problem with the word fasting is that people misinterpret it. It is not dieting or starving yourself. It is conditioning your body to properly channelizing the energy. It sends the right signals to various glands that they need to work properly. Your short fasting routines will help them in the job.

If you are resolute about trimming that belly fat and want to make yourself, more energetic, then intermittent fasting is the way to go for you. You will start noticing a visible change in your energy levels within a short span of few weeks. You can speed things up with exercise and healthy diet. Every effort that you make will complement weight loss.

This book will explain the correct way to do intermittent fasting. It will explain-

- ✓ The fact-based scientific approach towards fasting

- ✓ The difference in results between frequent eating and intermittent fasting

- ✓ The advantages of intermittent fasting

- ✓ The results you can expect

- ✓ The various methods that can be used without interrupting your normal life

There are plenty of books on this subject on the market, thanks again for choosing this one! Every effort was made to ensure it is full of as much useful information as possible, please enjoy!

Chapter 1: Understanding Intermittent Fasting and Some Related Misconceptions

✓ **Analyzing High-Frequency Meals**

Forming ideas based on common practice is not uncommon. In fact, it is natural to adopt methods that are convenient and then protect them as God's truth. This has happened with the idea of frequent eating too. Ask people in general, and they would unanimously support the idea that eating smaller meals at regular interval. They will vouch for its effectiveness with strong arguments. They'll go to say that It helps in weight loss and keeps the body energized. You can find scores of people that would vehemently discard the idea of fasting and dieting. But, have you ever tried to find the scientific basis of both the ideas?

In general, the nutritionists advise that eating 6 meals a day keeps your metabolism high. It stops you from hitting the metabolic plateau known as the starvation mode. But, in reality, there hasn't been one study to substantiate these claims. These are the claims originating out of occupational loyalty. The job of a nutritionist is to keep you well fed and nourished. This advice suits their job description which is to keep you well fed and nourished. But, making you lose your belly fat and bring it in shape isn't necessarily their responsibility. Several misconceptions cloud the thinking of medical professionals too. The hoax of six small meals in a day is one among them.

However, there are two types of problems in this theory. The first one is a practical problem. Suppose you start implementing six meals a day routine. You have the goal to either reduce, control or maintain your weight if not all. This means that-

- You will have to restrict your calorie intake to 2000

- Eat 6 times a day without eating more than 2000 calories

- You will have limited types of food you can eat

- Most food will increase the caloric intake

- The meals will get frugal and tasteless

- Food preparation time would increase a lot

- Storebought and packaged foods would become off limit. (They aren't advisable anyhow)

Now, the practical problem is that it isn't a sustainable solution for full-time moms. As a full-time mom, you have responsibilities. A job that you can't delegate to anyone else. Duties that you need to complete on time, every day. It isn't like being late for an office presentation. Your missing a responsibility can mean your kids missing school or performing badly in school. It may even result in bitterness in the family environment. So, time and routine aren't in your favor here. This will require elaborate preparation. Preparing 6 meals a day in place of 3 is more demanding. Following it up regularly may get difficult. You not only have to prepare more meals now but also have to ensure that they do not cross the calorie barrier.

There are technical problems too. There is a lack of studies that corroborate the success of this method. The major portion of this urban myth comes from uncertified sources. Largely from cereal and breakfast marketing advertisements and taglines. Frequent meals will become very difficult to regulate. In fact, a study conducted to find out the '*Effects of Increased Meal Frequency on Fat Oxidation, and Perceived Hunger*' found quite the opposite. It states that increasing meal frequency from three to six a day has no effect on fat oxidation. Our body would burn the same amount of calories in processing the food. However, it did find that there has been a significant increase in hunger and desire to eat in high-frequency meals. You will end up consuming more calories. Even your insulin resistance may increase. So, if you intend to control your weight, then this methodology is definitely not going to work for you.

✓ Effect of Intermittent Fasting on Weight Loss

The biggest argument given against intermittent fasting is that it sends wrong signals to the body. People say that fasting sends the body into starvation mode. The body would slow down the metabolic activities. In principle, this is true. If the body realizes that it is starving it would start conserving energy and lower the metabolic rate. But, the truth ends here. It takes at around 72-96 hours for the starvation mode to set in after your last meal. Intermittent fasting is a food interval of 14-24 hours at the most. It cannot send your body into a starvation mode in any case. On the contrary, studies have shown that the metabolic rate actually increases between 3.6%-14% after short-term fasting. This happens as our body frantically searches for energy sources and starts breaking down stored fat. Fat oxidation speeds up during this period. Our body has learned it from evolutionary practice. It has been the survival trick throughout the evolutionary history.

Our body, like other systems, follows a hierarchy system when it comes to energy consumption. It tries to burn the easiest form of energy available at first, i.e. blood sugar and glycogen. When that energy is exhausted, it switches to difficult forms of energy like fat deposits. Now, when we eat at frequent intervals, there is plenty of easy energy in the form of blood sugar and glycogen. The body never needs to use the fat deposits. Slowly and gradually the formation of enzymes that help in burning body fat lowers. The blood sugar and glycogen levels only come down when our body has been in a fasting state for 8-12 hours. Only then our body would start burning the body fat. If you want to reduce your body fat and trim your belly, then intermittent fasting for at least 14 hours is the best way to do so. This book will tell you the ways you can do it easily. You will also get to know the advantages of doing so and the scientific basis for those.

Chapter 2: Intermittent Fasting- The Real Deal

Obesity has emerged as an epidemic. The alarming thing is, there has been a steep rise in obesity rates among women. A study published in *Times health* states that the obesity rate was 40% among women in the US as compared to 35% in the men. The worrying fact is that it has become constant among men, but it is still rising among women year on year. The study noted an increase of 3% in a span of two years from 2014 -2016.

The ill effects of obesity are well known to everyone and need not be stressed out. Obesity has become the leading cause of diseases causing deaths in the US. Heart diseases, hypertension, osteoarthritis, and metabolic issues are some of the major problems. The more surprising fact is that most people in the US know about it. However, there is still a dearth of effective steps.

176

Popular Weight loss measures and the reasons for their ineffectiveness

- **Dieting**

The experiments with dieting have been the favored national timepass. Dieting has been a billion dollar industry. Too many variations and tricks and yet the results have been unimpressive. The major reason is the lack of established methodologies. Dieting is difficult to follow, time taking and needs very strict discipline. Frankly speaking, it is difficult to follow in the current fast-paced life. Stating a UCLA research, Associate professor of psychology in UCLA, Tracl Mann said that the people who lost 5-10% of their weight through diet regained it fast. He said that sustaining the weight loss was very difficult through dieting. He also said that between one-third to two-thirds people on diet regain more weight that they actually lost.

- **Exercise**

The exercise, yoga, and similar fitness regimen can undoubtedly bring good results. But, the instance you fall out of the routine, you'll start gaining weight at an even faster pace. For all practical reasons, this even makes exercise unfavorable as the first choice.

- **Surgery**

When all fails people turn towards medicine. Medical science has made significant progress. Several bariatric procedures boast of controlling weight. One such procedure touted greatly was gastric banding. However, slowly people realized that maintaining the lost weight is really difficult. People gained the lost weight pretty soon, and the whole exercise went in vain. Other procedures have also shown somewhat similar results. The cost is high, the risk is great, but the gain is inconsistent. This makes even the bariatric surgeries a less favored option. To make matters worse, most people wouldn't agree to go under the knife for weight reduction. To add salt to the misery, it is not only very expensive but getting the approval of doctors and insurance companies is also tricky.

Intermittent Fasting- The Time-tested Solution

When all else fails, we tend to look towards nature. The answer has always been there. We always knew the answer as our ancestors have been practicing it for centuries. It lay in their eating practice. Our ancestors were nomads. The probability of finding food was low for them. So, the fasting periods were frequent. This is the key to burning fat. Although it is true that our body slows the metabolic rate after it starts fearing starvation, but that doesn't happen very soon. Before the starvation mode, our body is frantically searching for energy sources to fuel survival efforts. Our body draws this energy from the fat deposits in our body. This is the key to our quest. If we can make our body look for energy sources more often then it will start burning fat deposits and help in trimming that belly fat.

Some of the striking features of Intermittent Fasting are:

- It is an easy and sustainable way to maintain weight for full-time moms

- It doesn't require extensive preparation

- You wouldn't need to take out time every now and then to eat

- You can go on with your normal routine most of the day

- The greater part of fasting would take place at night when you aren't active.

The reason Intermittent Fasting is highly effective in the long-run:

- It is easy to adhere to Intermittent Fasting in the long run- Sustainability

- It doesn't interfere with what you eat

- You get your nutritional requirements

- It accelerates fat loss but not the loss of lean body mass

- It is easy to apply and monitor

- It is safe for long-term practice and has proven results

- You can do it without any external help

- Supplementing it with exercise and dietary changes will help in rapid weight loss

Most Important

It reduces Insulin Resistance. It is the single most important factor in reducing the risk of most chronic diseases. It can reduce the risk of problems like type 2 diabetes, cardiovascular diseases, strokes, and cancer.

The best thing about intermittent fasting is that it is very easy to implement. You naturally spend 7-8 hours without eating anything at night. This is the time you are sleeping. Extending this time by few more hours will not only boost your weight loss efforts but will also give added benefits.

Studies have proved that intermittent fasting can help in balancing your cholesterol levels. It significantly reduces the risk of heart diseases. Your blood coagulation profile also improves greatly. This helps in reducing the risk of blood clots and strokes. The risk of chronic inflammation also decreases significantly.

This is important to make it clear from the outset that fasting is different from dieting. Dieting is being selective about the kind of food that you can eat. You go on a calorie restrictive diet. You become picky about the things to eat and the amount in which you'll eat them.

Intermittent fasting is all about bringing a change in the eating pattern. You do not spread out your meals throughout your day. You get a limited eating window. For men, the ideal intermittent fasting period lasts for 16 hours. For women, a 14 hour fasting period is enough. Once your fasting ends, you can eat. You can eat the same amount of food in two or three meals within the remaining 8-10 hours of the day.

You will not need to make any change in your daily schedule. You would not need to do lengthy meal preparations. An exercise routine in the morning before ending the daily fast would help immensely. However, its absence wouldn't cause any negative impact.

You can boost your weight loss efforts by being selective about the things you eat. If you do not eat too many excess calories in a day, it will help. We are what we eat, and it will always remain true. You can go a long way by remaining conscious of the things you eat. However, there are no restrictions.

The fasting period doesn't restrict your fluid intake. You can drink water or sugar-free beverages. The main emphasis is to give your body time to start burning the fat deposits in your body instead of glucose.

The health benefits of Intermittent Fasting are:

- Rapid fat burning and weight loss
- Increased HGH production
- Improvement of beneficial gut bacteria
- Improved Leptin Sensitivity
- Ghrelin Hormone normalization
- Improved tolerance of Glucose
- Metabolism Boost
- A better appreciation of food
- A fixed routine
- Enhanced brain function

- Better immune system
- Glowing skin
- Improved spiritual consciousness
- Lower oxidative stress

The best thing about Intermittent Fasting, it is possible to follow the routine even for full-time moms. You can do it without sacrificing any of your roles. It gives you complete flexibility. You'd remain free from the guilt pangs of dieting. You will have your cheat days. You will be able to enjoy your life better. You would look better without having to rely on external sources. This is the best measure to improve your health. If those tummy tires are making you conscious, start it. If you want to make your body slim and trim, start it. Take one step towards healthy living and give yourself and your family one more reason to smile. Because, you may feel it or not, but you are the engine of this train.

Intermittent fasting will keep you going and help you in staying fit even without making desperate efforts.

The following chapters would explain the scientific basis of the advantages mentioned above.

Chapter 3: Fat Burning and Weight Loss

Intermittent fasting is a natural concept for many communities around the world. They eat before sunset and do not eat for many hours after sunrise. This promotes good health. However, this practice comes to them in the form of religious practices and rituals. But, this doesn't undermine the positive impact of the practice. A religion called Jainism in India strongly promotes this practice.

It is important to look a bit deeper into the roots to understand the need for this practice.

Jain community is a trading community. Majority of the followers of this religion have been shopkeepers, traders, and businesspersons. Longer hours of sitting and sedentary lifestyle made the accumulation of fat easy. Being a wealthy community, they had no scarcity of rich food and that also added to the weight. This has been going on for centuries. The elders in the community must have realized this and understood the root of the problem. That's why, as a ritual, the followers of this religion do not eat after sunset. They can only eat hours after sunrise, and this means a gap of more than 16 hours. This intermittent fasting routine helps them in using up the fat.

This age-old practice is a testimony to the success of this principle. It shows the tried and tested results and efficacy of the routine.

Now, let's understand its functioning and the impact on fat burning and weight loss.

As explained earlier, our body will burn easy sources of energy first. The glucose and glycogen come in this category. It would have been fine if you had been consuming the same amount of calories you burnt. But, that's not possible in principle. You will become energy deficient. Your body keeps storing some energy in form of fat deposits for the rainy days. Therefore, when you eat, the consumed food gives out glucose and glycogen. The glucose gets dissolved in the blood directly. The body loves to use this energy. It is the blood sugar, and it is very easy to break. Then our body uses the glycogen, which remains deposited in our liver. Each meal can keep releasing this glucose up to 8 hours. This means that if you are eating six meals a day, your body will never get a chance to lay hands upon the fat deposits. Because it is getting easy energy supply in plenty. You are replenishing the deposits much faster than they are needed. This is the cause of the problem.

When you begin intermittent fasting, your body stops getting the easily available glucose. In that case, it has to start burning the fat deposits. The fat deposits are difficult to burn. But, they provide a great amount of energy. The energy thus produced is sustainable. You may start feeling lower appetite. Your consumption of energy may also reduce. This speeds up your weight loss efforts.

Studies have also proved that once you start intermittent fasting your urge to eat continuously vanishes. You feel more satiated. You will not feel energy deprived or weak because you are still getting the sufficient amount of calories per day. You are just depriving your body of easy fuel for a certain period. It has a very positive impact on your weight loss efforts. This leads to faster fat burning and weight loss. As a full-time mom, you can't ask for things to get better.

You can choose the fasting schedule of your choice. It just needs to be 14 hours long. You can choose to start your fast at 6 in the evening. Get up at 6 or 7 in the morning as per your convenience and do your exercise routine. Have your breakfast at 8 eight and things would be sorted. This isn't a difficult routine to follow as after eating at 6 it is unlikely to feel hungry by 9 or 10. If you sleep early, then it can be ideal for you. However, if you follow another schedule, then you can make the adjustments accordingly.

Following a fixed schedule would be easy. You may feel hungry in the beginning, but you'll get used to it very quickly. This will make intermittent fasting a part of your normal life. You can lose weight and stop gaining it without extra efforts.

Several experiments conducted on rats and mice show that intermittent fasting fared better in weight loss. Even with the same amount of calorie intake, the rats on intermittent fasting lost significant weight.

The good thing is that you can carry on with your intermittent fasting for the whole week and take weekends as cheat days. This prevents the schedule from coming in the way of your regular life. You can enjoy your family get-togethers without guilt pangs.

It increases the benefits of exercise

If you are trying to get faster results, exercise during the fasting period is the best. There is a simple reason behind this. In the 14-16 hour fasting state there is no blood sugar or glycogen as the easy energy source. When you burn energy your body will have to derive that from your fat deposits.

You can lose 3-8% of your body weight within 3-24 weeks. It may also lead to a reduction of your waist circumference to the tune of 4-7%.

Chapter 4: Reduce Waist Circumference by Improving Insulin Sensitivity

Insulin is one of the most important hormones released by our body. It plays a vital role in our lives, and almost half of all metabolic and lifestyle problems in the modern world are due to insulin imbalance. In simple words, insulin is the power broker hormone. Its main job is to bind with cells and help them absorb the blood glucose and other energy sources. Low insulin secretion can cause severe energy crisis in the body, and the system may begin to shut down. Insulin imbalance can cause diabetes and other metabolic issues too.

Our body has a very swift and sophisticated system of energy absorption. The glucose from all kind of food items starts to dissolve in the blood whenever we eat. Our body senses the increase in blood glucose and gives instructions to our pancreas to release insulin. It can bind to your cells and help them in absorbing this glucose. They'll then be able to use it as a direct energy source. Without insulin, the blood sugar levels will keep increasing alarmingly, but our body will not get any energy. Insulin not only helps in burning the energy in form of glucose but it also assists our body in storing the excess sugar in form of fat. It constantly regulates the amount of sugar present in your blood. Till this point everything is good. The problem is in the excess.

Earlier, our ancestors struggled for every meal. They were energy deficient and hence whenever they consumed food it was swiftly broken into energy. Today, it is the age of convenience and excess. In the modern world, an abundance of food sources is common. You can eat whenever you like. Frequent snacking and munching has become a norm. This keeps the blood sugar levels spiked for the most part of the day. It is the point where the real problem begins.

Frequent meals keep the blood sugar levels high and in turn, lead to the constant release of insulin. The high amount of energy converted is not required for instant use. It leads to accumulation of unwanted fat. You are giving way to obesity. Having one energy bar here and a Popsicle there doesn't seem much, but in reality, it is. The constant release of insulin can make our cells develop insulin resistance. This means that there will be a high quantity of blood sugar and insulin in the blood, but our body will not be utilizing any of it. You would develop hyperinsulinemia leading to hyperglycemia. You'd stop burning any kind of fat, and the obesity will rise to the next level.

Insulin resistance is an alarming condition. Sadly, it is becoming a stark reality with 40% of US population getting affected by the condition. It is spreading its roots faster among the kids too.

Poor diet and insulin resistance leads to accumulation of visceral fat. The waist circumference keeps on increasing adding on fat tires around your belly. Research has proved that intermittent fasting can help in this scenario. A study conducted by Journal of Laboratory and Clinical Medicine showed that women on intermittent fasting can reduce 3-7% of their waist circumference through it. Intermittent fasting helps in improving your lipid profile and also improves insulin sensitivity. Here, it is important to note that better insulin sensitivity is opposite of insulin resistance. Your body will be able to process the blood sugar better.

It is a great solution for full-time moms riddled with insulin resistance. They can practice intermittent fasting and bring their belly fat under control.

Chapter 5: Human Growth Hormone (hGH)

Human Growth Hormone (hGH) has gained great recognition in the recent past. It has become a favorite of the people interested in bodybuilding or competitive sports. The reason for the interest is simple. It is a very powerful hormone with great benefits. It is a performance-enhancing hormone. It can give a great boost to your bodybuilding efforts. It promotes fitness, muscle growth, and longevity. It is also a hormone that can speed up your fat loss efforts. But, our body produces it in low quantities after teenage. People turn to synthetic hGH for getting these benefits. However, taking synthetic hGH injections without the supervision of experts is very dangerous. The US government has declared its sale and use illegal without a medical prescription. The same is the case with most governments in the world.

Our body stops producing hGH in large quantities once we cross the teenage. This is because the growth needs subside. However, our body still produces hGH in low quantities. Here, it will be important to understand the relation of hGH with another hormone called insulin. Our pancreas release insulin to transport sugar to our cells. The release of hGH can only take place when there is no presence of insulin in our blood. Until there is the presence of glucose, insulin secretion will continue. This will only stop after 8 hours of our food intake. By that time, our body uses all the freely available glucose. After that, Insulin production will halt, and our body can release hGH. Intermittent fasting can help you here. It allows the time for your body to release hGH as fasting spans are longer.

hGH secretion is usually high during three periods:

1. When you are sleeping

2. When you engage in high-intensity physical training

3. In case of trauma

Intermittent fasting prepares the ground for the release of hGH in ample quantities. This hormone can increase metabolic rate and aid fat loss. This important hormone is also vital for healing, growth, and repair of muscles. It aids protein synthesis. It is very important for increasing libido.

A research conducted by the team of Intermountain Medical Center Heart Institute found that intermittent fasting raised the levels of hGH secretion in women by 1300% and in men by 2000%. This can override all other benefits offered by intermittent fasting. hGH not only helps in cutting fat faster but it also has many other health benefits. It boosts immunity and helps the production of anabolic hormones too.

This will give you a definitive edge in your weight loss efforts. You will have natural hGH as performance enhancer without having to worry about the harmful effects or the costs. As a full-time mom, it doesn't take a lot to implement this is your life. A little bit of care and effort will give you the body you had been longing for since ages. All this comes without sacrificing the happiness of anyone.

Chapter 6: Bring Your Insatiable Hunger Under Control

Hunger is one of the strongest feelings in all beings. It is important for survival, and it keeps us going. It has been the most important reason for evolution. It keeps us going. It compels us to eat when we need energy the most. But, what if the hunger response goes into an overdrive? What if we keep feeling hungry all the time? Even imagining the result isn't pleasant.

However, it is a reality for most of the people suffering from obesity. They have an insatiable urge to eat and keep eating. Their hunger response is not out of necessity but due to a malfunction, and this is unhealthy. When you always feel hungry, you eat. Your body is not able to use that amount of energy, and it starts storing it as visceral fat. You start getting obese, and it gives way to new diseases. One thing leads to another, and the vicious cycle of diseases starts.

To control this insatiable hunger, it is important to understand the cause first. Our stomach releases a hormone called Ghrelin when its empty. It is a signal to our brain to start eating. Once you have eaten the required amount of food, the release of ghrelin hormone reduces. It is highest when your stomach is empty, and it completely stops after an hour of your eating. The substantial difference of this hormone in the two situations helps the brain to differentiate between the need to eat or not. The problem arises when your stomach keeps releasing ghrelin in small quantities all the time. It often happens with obese people. Their ghrelin release is never very high either they are empty stomach or full. This confuses the brain, and it doesn't think that you are full. You always have the urge to eat, and it adds more weight.

It is also important to note that ghrelin hormone also has another important function. It helps in the release of growth hormone. The longer you are hungry, the stronger is the release of hGH. As you know that hGH helps in the faster burning of fat, it is important to sustain the release of ghrelin. Eating would lower the release of ghrelin, and you would burn calories slower.

So, it is important that your body releases a high amount of ghrelin when you are empty stomach and stops its release once you are full. It is also helpful that you utilize the release of ghrelin for higher production of hGH.

Intermittent fasting helps you a lot in both. It helps in improving ghrelin sensitivity. Prolonged breaks between meals help in making your brain more sensitive to ghrelin. Your appetite gets regulated. Apart from that, the extended time taken before meal leads to the higher amount of ghrelin release. This, in turn, helps in the higher release of hGH. So, you not only eat the restricted amount of food, but you also start burning it more effectively. The constant hunger pangs subside, and things start to normalize. You will be able to shed weight better and trim that belly fat. Regulated food consumption doesn't lead to the accumulation of visceral fat. Your waist circumference would come under control.

Intermittent fasting will help you in controlling one of the biggest enemies of weight loss, constant craving for food.

However, you must also note that you will have to work a lot towards this goal. Ghrelin release is also affected by the kind of food you eat. The higher amount of processed sugar you will eat, the greater amount of ghrelin imbalance will occur. Processed sugar like fructose is difficult to break, and it leads to accumulation of visceral fat. You must eat healthy fiber-rich food and avoid processed food items that contain fructose.

You can go a long way in your goal of reducing weight and trimming your belly fat by controlling your diet. You must eat healthy food, do regular exercise along with intermittent fasting and the results would be phenomenal.

Chapter 7: Improve Leptin Sensitivity

We all know that there is a direct relationship between eating and weight gain. It is a no-brainer. The more you'll eat, the higher the amount of energy you'll get. You'll keep gaining weight. Our body has a check and balance system to keep things under control. When your body becomes energy deficient, it sends signals to your brain to eat. You eat and gain energy, then your body releases a satiety hormone called 'Leptin.' It signals your brain to stop eating as you are full. It keeps your appetite under control. However, things turn sour when this hormone malfunctions.

Fat cells release leptin to send signals to your brain that you do not need to eat more. It fills you with satiety. However, inflammation in the fat cells can create an imbalance in the production of this hormone. Higher fat in the body will lead to the release of a greater amount of leptin. This may create leptin resistance. Although there may be a great amount of leptin floating around your brain, it may not recognize it. It will keep thinking that your body is devoid of energy and hence it must continue eating. It starts a vicious cycle which leads to higher weight gain. High level of leptin is very harmful. You will have an insatiable hunger. You will become lethargic and stop burning fat. This, in turn, will lead to more fat gain.

Although there are several reasons for this, inflammation in the fat cells is main. Reducing the levels of leptin in your blood can help in improving leptin sensitivity. Intermittent fasting can help you in this. When you switch to intermittent fasting, you are training your body to remain without food for extended periods. During this time the leptin levels in your blood will become stable. When you eat food, you start feeling satiated early. Adopting a healthy lifestyle, switching over to low-carb and high fiber diet and exercise will also help you in fighting this problem.

You must avoid processed food as it kills the gut bacteria and increases inflammation. Inflammation is one of the biggest reasons and hence you must focus on reducing it. Eating healthy food is the key here. Consume healthy fats that aid the building of hormones. Focus on improving the gut functioning. Do not overload your system with too much food. Regular exercise also helps a lot in reducing leptin resistance. Your focus must remain on improving your overall health.

Several studies have found that intermittent fasting is a good way to improve leptin sensitivity. It helps in fighting inflammation and also lowers the level of free fatty acids in the blood. These are the two key things that lead to leptin resistance. Better leptin sensitivity will naturally reduce your appetite, and you will feel better. Your calorie intake will go down, and you will become leaner over time.

While you are trying to bring down leptin resistance, it is important to bring down your sugar intake. Limiting your fructose and processed carbohydrates intake will help you.

Once your leptin sensitivity improves, you will start feeling better. Your sleep will improve, and you will start feeling more energetic.

Chapter 8: Counter Inflammation Before It Hits You

Inflammation is your body's natural response to any infection. It helps you and starts the remedial procedure. It is a part of your body's immune system. The problem begins when inflammation becomes chronic. Your body keeps fighting with an issue for very long and isn't able to resolve the problem. In that case, your own inflammation process starts acting against you. Inflammation can be very dangerous in such cases. The bigger problem is that such inflammations can be going on for years, unnoticed. You might not even get to know about them. However, their impact on your health can be very serious.

Unnatural weight gain can be a result of one such inflammation. It may also cause an imbalance in the release of leptin or ghrelin hormones. Inflammation in the fat cells can lead to such problems. This makes quick handling of the problem important.

Inflammation in itself is not a disease. However, not taking care of it in due time can lead to the development of several diseases. Some very high-risk issues like Alzheimer's disease, cancer, and heart problems are related to it. Being overweight or obese further adds to the problem.

It is very important that you take inflammation seriously and start taking precautions. Your diet plays a very important role in tackling inflammation. Poor diet is the biggest trigger for it. If you are too much dependent on processed food, unhealthy fats, sugar-laden diet, then there will always be high chances of inflammation. A sedentary lifestyle and stressful environment at home or workplace may add to it.

Inflammation not only leads to deteriorated health but it also leads to low morale. You feel stressed, tired, and irritated. The quality of life goes down. The bigger problem with inflammation is that medicines are a poor cure for it. Medicines will suppress the symptoms but will not cure the problem. Hence, it will keep building inside you.

Intermittent fasting can help you in fighting inflammation. Especially, the one affecting your brain. Our brain releases a special type of protein called BDNF (Brain-Derived Neurotrophic Factor). It is crucial for many important brain functions. It stimulates the production of new brain cells and encourages neuroplasticity. Inflammation decreases the level of BDNF production. It may lead to serious problems like a decrease in blood flow and oxygen to the brain. The neuroplasticity or the capacity of your brain to regrow may also decrease. Your memory, learning, and capacity of high thinking may get affected.

Higher production of BDNF will help you in losing weight. It will suppress your food intake by signaling your brain properly. It also increases metabolism that helps in losing weight. Therefore, reducing inflammation and boosting the BDNF production is a good way to lose weight. It will improve the sensitivity of the brain towards various signals.

As discussed above, inflammation is caused by several factors. Bad diet, sedentary lifestyle, stress, and obesity are among the chief causes. To counter inflammation, you must work on these issues seriously. Improving your diet and consuming healthy food is the first step. A study conducted by Laboratory of Neurosciences, National Institute of Aging, Baltimore found that intermittent fasting can help in reducing inflammation and increasing the production of BDNF. Intermittent fasting is very effective in reducing free androgen index, C-reactive protein levels, total and LDL cholesterol, triglycerides, blood pressure, oxidative stress and other inflammation markers. All these lead to inflammation. As the inflammation level goes down the production of BDNF increases.

Intermittent fasting with exercise is a great solution for reducing inflammation. It can not only help in reducing weight but will also assist you in living a healthy and problem free life.

Chapter 9: Intermittent Fasting- Definitely Doable

Now, we know the advantages intermittent fasting offers. It can help you in trimming your belly fat and get limitless energy. The question arises, is it doable? The answer to this lies within you. Any plan can only work when you put your heart and mind to it. Intermittent fasting is a way. In fact, it is one of the best and easiest ways to trim the belly fat. As a full-time mom, you have a lot of responsibilities. You have a lot of weight on your shoulders, and no one can fill in your shoes. But, your health is also important. The belly fat is just not a cosmetic problem, but it will also give rise to many serious health issues. If you want to remain in a position to look after your family like this for long, then you will have to take concrete steps. Increasing belly fat will not take you anywhere.

Intermittent fasting is the simplest and most effective solution you have. It doesn't come in the way of your daily life. It doesn't ask you to do extraordinary things. It doesn't take away your focus from your prime responsibility. It gives you limitless energy. It makes you regain your lost figure. It fills you with confidence. It gives you positive and spiritual energy. You will feel rejuvenated and good. So, the simple answer to the earlier question is a Yes.

However, success doesn't come without sacrifices. You will have to sacrifice some momentary pleasures. Self-control is the pre-requisite of intermittent fasting. You will have to control the urge to eat in the initial phase. Putting some control on the type of food you eat will help a lot. Intermittent fasting doesn't require you to go on a calorie deficient diet. It doesn't ask you to remove any kind of food from your menu. But, avoiding processed foods, unhealthy fats, and added sugar will boost your weight loss efforts. The same is with exercise. Intermittent fasting prepares the most fertile ground for burning fat quickly. The high amount of hGH produced during intermittent fasting will help you in rapidly losing weight. It will also help in positive regrowth of lost muscles. It starts a complete rejuvenation process. But, for that to take effect, you will have to put some extra effort in exercise. It isn't important to pump iron for hours or do rigorous weight training. Even light exercise will also help your body in mobilizing the body fat. All these steps are complementary to intermittent fasting. They will help your goal of shedding weight faster and feeling more energetic. However, they are not mandatory. You can begin with intermittent fasting first and then switch on to healthy food and exercise. The positive outcome will motivate you towards taking extra steps. You can move one step at a time.

Intermittent fasting is especially the best solution for full-time moms as it is practical. Dozens of time it happens that we make resolutions for weight loss. We swear that we'll do everything in our power to reduce the excess fat. We saddle up and even go for a rigorous routine. But soon the enthusiasm fades away and in place of it realization dawns upon us. We sense that we are faltering on our commitments. We feel that the routine is not working for us. We assess that the results are not satisfactory and hence we should stop punishing ourselves. Out of ordinary efforts seek extraordinary results, and failure to achieve that quickly can cause disappointment. Countering this problem is very important.

Intermittent fasting doesn't require extraordinary efforts. It doesn't push you to the limits. It doesn't seek extra time from you. You can practice with without being in the eyes of the world, and the results are fabulous.

All you need to do is choose an intermittent fasting plan that suits your lifestyle. Adjust it according to your needs. Once the transition is complete adopt extra measures like healthy food and exercise to supplement your efforts. The results will be better than your expectation. It is a high success approach towards weight loss, and it doesn't interfere with the daily affairs of your life. It gives you complete freedom and flexibility. You will have your cheat days, so you don't have to look abnormal or desperate. You can practice it without advertising to the whole world. No one needs to know if you don't want to tell.

Obesity and belly fat are big problems. They are among the major health risks these days. Our lifestyle and food are not helping us in any way either. Switching to a healthy lifestyle that helps us in fighting inflammation and diseases is important. Intermittent fasting will open your ways towards it.

The next chapter will explain several intermittent fasting plans to choose from. Pick a plan that suits you the best and dedicate yourself to it. Put your heart and mind to it. You will see a visible change in yourself in a very short span.

Chapter 10: Intermittent Fasting Plans

Intermittent fasting keeps your stomach empty for long periods. You can make that happen in any way you like. You can do this irrespective of your lifestyle. You can choose the time and plan as per your liking. Even in the same plan, you can create variations. The end goal is to remain in a fasted state for an extended period. However, it is always beneficial to follow a specific plan to get the best and fastest results. There are some common intermittent fasting plans followed all over the globe. You can choose the one you like the most. The only important thing is to stick to it and follow it properly. Eat healthy while you are at it and break free from the sedentary lifestyle. Exercise along with intermittent fasting will fetch you superb results.

1. Daily Intermittent Fasting Plan

This is the easiest and most convenient fasting plan. It is easy to follow and implement. In this plan, the fasting period is of 14 hours for women and 16 hours for men. So, if you are a full-time mom, this plan will work like magic for you. It is the least stressful and takes minimal effort. You will have a 10-hour eating window which is suitable for 2-3 meals. You will just need to shift one meal ahead to accommodate this plan.

If you are a morning person and avoiding breakfast for long can be a problem, then you can begin this fast early in the evening. The night makes it easier to keep the hunger pangs aside. In case you remain awake till late at night you can begin the fast a bit late in the evening and skip your breakfast to finish the fasting time. The goal is to complete 14 hours of the fasting period.

To understand it in clear terms let us break the schedule. For example, if you choose to begin the fast early in the evening, you can finish your last meal of the day at around 5. Your fasting state would last around 7 in the morning. You can do your normal exercise routine before this time. You can easily have your breakfast and begin your day as normal. This plan would work best for all the moms who need to wake up early. You will have a 10-hour window till 5 in the evening to distribute your 2-3 meals of the day as per your convenience. In a few days time, you will get habitual of the plan and wouldn't feel even the slightest of craving for food in the fasted state. The best thing about this schedule is that you will have a very short window to feel the craving. After eating at 5 in the evening, you wouldn't feel hungry for the next few hours. In the morning you can have your breakfast early, and hence you wouldn't have to subside your hunger for long.

In case, you stay awake for long at night and feel that you might get hungry after eating at 5 then you can shift your last meal ahead. However, you must remember that eating your last meal 2-3 hours prior to your bedtime is important. It helps in proper digestion of food and keeps you healthy. So, if you have your last meal at 9, then you will have to stay in the fasted state until eleven the next day. This means that you will have to skip your breakfast. If this schedule suits you, then you can go for it as well.

Your focus must remain on few simple things. This is a daily intermittent fasting plan, and hence it brings consistency. You don't have to remember days, time and things like that. The fasting becomes a natural part of your life, and hence the transition is easy. But, in the beginning, you will have to put extra effort to maintain the consistency. There can be days when you fail to follow the schedule, but that must not deter you from trying the next day.

You must maintain an active lifestyle. Exercise is the best, but if you are not up for it in the beginning, then you must at least try brisk walks and strolls. This will utilize the production of hGH in your body. Your fat would get metabolized faster, and you would get better results.

Adopting intermittent fasting in your lifestyle is a signal that you want a positive change in your life. You want to get rid of the extra weight you are carrying. You want to remain fit and fabulous. Shedding unhealthy food is also a part of it. Your food is important. It can help you in staying healthy and fit. You do not need to discard everything at once. But, you must begin. Start by removing processed food from your diet. Add more fiber and whole grain foods. Eat healthy fats that have lots of antioxidants. This will give you a new lease on life.

This plan is the best for full-time moms as it isn't disruptive. It fits into your daily routine like a hand in glove. You do not have to distract yourself from your routine life. Extra efforts and precaution in food can fetch excellent results. You will start losing weight fast, and the positive effects of intermittent fasting go much beyond that. It will give you positive energy. You will feel happier and connected. It is easy to adopt even for beginners and works like a charm for the experienced ones too.

2. The 5:2 Plan

This intermittent fasting plan allows you to eat normal diet on five days of the week and you can fast on two days of your choice. However, unlike the daily intermittent fasting plans, you cannot eat normal diet on the fasting days. You will have to restrict your calorie intake to 500 calories. This plan has several positive and negative things which we will discuss now.

To start with the positive aspects of this diet, it is very effective. A study published in Journal of Diabetes and Vascular Diseases states that this is a very effective strategy for weight loss. It also says that this fasting helps in improving important parameters like insulin sensitivity and health biomarkers.

Let us first understand how it works. You can choose two days of your choice for this type of fasting. Weekdays are preferable as they keep your weekends free for social get together and outings.

You can choose to indulge yourself in those days. However, on the days of your fast, you are only allowed to consume 500 calories during the eating window. This plan may look a bit tough, but it isn't impractical. But, it would definitely take more effort to adopt as it would not become a part of the habit.

This plan would require a lot of self-control as the meals are going to be small. Living on paltry 500 calories for a day can be tough for some people, and you may feel odd in the beginning. However, you can get used to it and reap the benefits of the plan. Studies have shown that this type of diet gives similar results to continuous calorie restriction. You will lose weight fast, and there will be an improvement in the insulin sensitivity and other health biomarkers.

However, when going for such plans, it is important to treat the phrase 'normal diet' with caution. When you are trying to lose weight, it is important to keep your normal diet and eating frequency under control. Besides few cheat days, you must pay attention to what you and the quantities in which you eat.

As for the negative aspects of this diet, it is a bit tough. You should begin with daily intermittent fasting and when you get accustomed to it, then only switch to this. It is difficult to get used to this fasting style as there is lack of continuity. But, your body slowly gets used to the calorie restricted fasting schedule of 24 hours.

3. Alternate Day Intermittent Fasting Plan

This method takes intermittent fasting to the next level. It is like increasing the difficulty level of a video game. However, the rewards are also equally high.

In this fasting plan, you will have to fast every other day. You can choose the type of fast you want to keep. This means that you can choose to eat 500 calorie diet in the ten-hour eating window or abstain from eating completely. The choice will be completely yours. This kind of fasting regimen is a bit extreme and should only be tried once you have got habitual of fasting. This plan has its own advantages. You go low on calorie intake and hence losing weight becomes easy. Insulin sensitivity and other health biomarkers improve considerably.

This is a difficult method. It may look disruptive as going hungry for a full day, every other day can be difficult. It can put a lot of strain. You may feel less energetic on your fasting days in the beginning. As for the benefits, there are plenty. Low-calorie intake expedites the fat loss. It improves insulin sensitivity. The hGH formation increases and helps you in muscle formation and weight loss. But, this plan is not for everyone. It should only be tried once you have got accustomed to the previous two plans.

4. Warrior Diet

This diet excessively focuses on a correct diet along with a strict intermittent fasting plan. If you are not determined enough or feel that you can go on with moderate efforts, then this isn't for you. This diet requires the practitioners to remain on a strict food plan where they can only eat some raw fruits and vegetables in the day. They will only get a 4-hour eating window in which they can have a full meal. The day diet only consists of small amounts of raw fruits and vegetables. It pushes you to the limits as this is not a once in a week occurrence. This will become a routine. It strictly removes all unhealthy fats and processed food items from your diet. You will also have to avoid grains, meats, refined foods as well as products laden with artificial sugar.

This diet plan is difficult to follow. It would take a lot of effort to get accustomed to this diet. However, the results would be astonishing. It is called a warrior diet because it prepares you like one. This has been the eating pattern of human beings throughout the evolutionary history. It has made us survive against all the odds. It not only targets excess fat but also improves your overall health biomarkers. This diet will reduce all kinds of chronic inflammations and reduce oxidative stress. The combination of right diet and fasting can spell magic for you. It will work more effectively than any other form of intermittent fasting. The reason is simple, it cuts not only your eating time but also the kind of food you eat. You consume fewer fats and carbs. You eat more fiber that helps your gut environment. You can get free from most of the problems. But, if you are just starting the intermittent fasting regimen, then jumping directly to this plan can be a mistake. It would require immense self-control and practice. You must move ahead step by step. Once you get habitual of restricted diet then only you should proceed to this diet.

All these intermittent fasting plans are there to help you with your weight loss goals. But, their advantage is just not limited to it. It will improve your overall health and give you limitless energy. All you need to do is to stick to any of the plans and follow it religiously. Not being sincere enough will fetch poor results. To make it a long-term effort it is also important to work in an organized manner. Do not jump the steps or get over enthusiastic. Always remember that slow and steady wins the race.

Intermittent fasting is a great solution to a big problem. Weight loss has been a billion dollar industry. Obesity is spreading like an epidemic, and it is causing a score of other problems too. Keeping the weight under check is important to remain safe. Intermittent fasting can help you in that if you follow it properly. It is a great way to reduce weight and cut the belly fat for full-time moms. You can practice it within the four walls of your home. All you would need is will and self-control.

Chapter 11: How Should You Approach It

The best way to approach anything is to approach it positively. Again, the saying slow and steady wins the race is important here. Being overzealous about such things can cause problems. People start their efforts with full force and begin losing motivation very soon when they see the results are not according to their expectation. You can't rush the process. You are acting against your own body. Use of brute force is not good. You'd end up becoming a spent force very soon.

When it comes to full-time moms the situation gets even trickier. You have a world of responsibilities. Rushing with weight loss programs can not only have poor but adverse results too. Intermittent fasting is a very steady approach towards weight loss with proven results. It is a complete transformation technique practiced all around the world. It will not only help you in reducing the belly fat and weight but will also help you psychologically and spiritually. You would become stronger and positive.

The biggest concern of the beginners is about their success. You may be hesitant that it will be difficult to follow. You may be absolutely correct. But, you'd never know it without ever trying once. There are no fallouts of failing. There is no public shame. On the positive side, there is a high probability that you wouldn't fail. Start with the easy process and stick to it. There might be some hunger pangs. You might feel your stomach gurgling. But, you have all the time, liberty and freedom to adjust the timings as per your convenience. This reduces the chances of failure in your efforts. You just need to stay calm. You can drink water, tea or coffee or any other non-caloric beverages during the fasting time. It will reduce the effect of hunger. Over time, these issues will subside and your body will adjust itself to this positive change.

Intermittent fasting in itself can also work as a standalone solution. However, its effectiveness would reduce when you keep stuffing yourself with unhealthy food. What you eat plays a very important role. Sticking to a good diet is very important. There are some things that you must avoid as much as possible. Then there are others that you need to increase.

Good Food:

Healthy fats: Like good and bad bacteria there is good and bad fat. Healthy fats are full of antioxidants and reduce oxidative stress. Carbohydrates and Sugar: Carbohydrate and sugar are the main energy sources. However, you should remain cautious about the kind of sugar you are consuming. The glucose in fruits is sweet and healthy. But, the refined sugar you eat is not. You must reduce the intake of refined sugar and increase the consumption of fruits and vegetables.

Probiotics: Gut health is very important. It can keep the danger of inflammation in control. It will improve your immunity and improve digestion. You should consume probiotic food in high quantity.

Food items to avoid:

Processed Foods: These foods contain a lot of sugar. They harm your gut bacteria and help in causing inflammation. These food items cause fat accumulation and will spike your insulin levels.

Unhealthy Fats: Refined and hydrogenated fats like vegetable oils can cause a lot of problems. They lead to fat accumulation and cause free radical damage. They are a leading cause of oxidative stress. You must avoid the use of unhealthy fats.

You should include the good things in your diet and keep your calorie intake under check. Regular exercise in any form is also very helpful. You will get the best results through it.

So, if you are just stepping into intermittent fasting, then there is no reason to rush already. You should start one thing at a time and then include other healthy things into the routine. The important thing is to try to make it a natural part of your daily life. Forming a habit of the routine will bring consistency, and you wouldn't have to put extra efforts. Intermittent fasting brings great results, and you wouldn't be disappointed by it. The important thing is to take the plunge and begin it.

Chapter 12: A Word of Caution

Intermittent fasting is a serious commitment, and it has sound results. However, sometimes even good things can interfere with existing conditions. Hence, it is important that you consider those before beginning intermittent fasting.

Intermittent fasting is not advisable for pregnant and breastfeeding mothers. The reason is very simple. They need more nutrition. Their baby is dependent on the food they are eating. If they deprive themselves of proper food, then it may affect the health of their baby. They can always shed the extra pounds of pregnancy fat at any later stage.

If you are anemic and underweight or suffering from any kind of eating disorder, then you shouldn't do it. Intermittent fasting deprives you of regular nutrition, and that can be dangerous in such conditions. Always ask your physician before beginning any such fasting schedule.

The only visible side effect of intermittent fasting is hunger. You may feel hungry, weak and light headed. But, there are no reasons to worry as these are temporary symptoms. Your body is trying to switch the energy sources from readily available glucose to fat. It will help you in the long run. This hunger will actually help you in remaining energetic and increase your fat processing abilities.

One very important thing to remember is that once you break your fast practice self-control. People generally start making elaborate meal plans before ending their fasts. Eating heavy after a fast can cause acidity and discomfort. Start the day with a lighter meal. You can have a second heavy meal after some time. Do not be in a haste. Remember that your goal is to lose weight. Gorging too much food will be a problem to that goal. This self-control will be more important in the beginning. Once you get accustomed to the schedule, your hunger will subside. The desire to eat more goes down with intermittent fasting, and you naturally feel less hungry.

But, you must get an expert medical opinion before beginning intermittent fasting if you are suffering from any of the following:

- Diabetes

- Blood Pressure

- Blood Sugar Problems

- Underweight

- Anemic

- Taking Treatment for Some Other Medical Condition

- If You are Trying to Conceive

- Have a History of Amenorrhea

- Pregnant or Breastfeeding

Apart from such medical constraints, you are free to practice intermittent fasting and get great results. This is a great way of losing weight for full-time moms. You can reap the benefits without going an extra mile. So, if you are fed up of those tummy tires tainting your figure, then go for it. It is a great solution for trimming that belly fat and getting limitless energy.

Book 4: Intermittent Fasting for Women

How to Lose Weight Without Impacting Your Social Life

By

Beatrice Anahata

Introduction

Congratulations on grabbing your copy of Intermittent Fasting for Women: How to Lose Weight Without Impacting Your Social Life and thank you for doing so.

The following chapters will discuss how you can safely intermittent fast with the method of your choice, while still enjoying an active social life. There are tips and tricks that help you fit intermittent fasting into your busy life without making sacrificing important social events.

There are plenty of books on this subject on the market, thanks again for choosing this one! Every effort was made to ensure it is full of as much useful information as possible, please enjoy!

Chapter 1: Finding the Right Fasting Method to Fit Into Your Lifestyle

You're busy living your life and for many people that can get in the way of making your health a priority. Sticking to a diet that involves counting calories or carbohydrates can often provide more stress into your already busy life. That's why so many people start and diet and quit, not because they didn't try, but because it actually makes their life harder. It's not a surprise that life can be overwhelming, everyone has been there. Dieting that involves constant number crunching and restricting is time consuming, and quite frankly, not good for mental health. No one wants to add more stress to their lives, especially about something as natural and important as eating, this is something you have been doing your entire life. So as your life gets busier, it might be better to use your busy schedule to adjust your eating behavior in a way that works for you.

As humans, we love food, and that's okay, a lot of our social lives even revolve around it. Think about how many times you go out with friends to have dinner, or how many times you are bombarded with commercials about food. You could imagine how difficult it would be to be faced with the task of counting all of the calories you are consuming. That could really take the fun out of eating, which with the stresses from normal day to day life, that's really the last thing you need. That's why so many people find themselves trying trendy or fad diets and then not succeeding because it is simply not feasible for everyone. Sometimes it is important to be able to enjoy a dessert, you've worked hard all week and feel like you deserve it. Intermittent fasting is not going to take that away from you.

This is why intermittent fasting is an alternative solution, you are not going to stop eating, you are just going to change the times in which you do. That means that you don't have to give up the foods you love, as a matter of fact, there is very little restricting involved at all. With intermittent fasting you're not changing what you eat, but when you eat. Many people hear the word 'fast' and assume that you are going to be starving. That could not be farther from the truth, think about how long you go without eating when you sleep, anywhere from 6 to 8 hours depending on how long you sleep. That doesn't mean you're starving, your body is already accustomed to going sometime without eating. Intermittent fasting gives you the ability to control your food intake in a way that fits into your life.

Most diets that require you to restrict calories or carbohydrates are a one-size-fits-all method. Diets like these have one right way to do everything, regardless of your body type, schedule, or lifestyle. That's not setting you up for success, it is the opposite, making it nearly impossible to succeed. Not everyone's life and schedule are the same and many diets do not take that into consideration. Intermittent fasting has many different methods for you to choose from and even more, you can also tweak these methods even more to make them even more personalized.

However, intermittent fasting is not a diet, it is more than that. It is a lifestyle change, meaning this is something that is going to affect more than just your diet. It requires some discipline and patience, but once you start, you are going to see results and actually want to continue. Intermittent fasting is one of the best ways to burn real fat, not just the loss of water weight like low carbohydrate diets. Your body will learn to burn fat stores as fuel, allowing you to lose weight and keep it off. This is why intermittent fasting has the ability to target stomach fat, since this is one of the most common areas people hold fat, therefore it is one of the first places that fat stores are reduced.

As mentioned above, there are many different methods when it comes to intermittent fasting. Some of them involve going longer periods without eating, known as the fasting period than others. One method doesn't involve fasting at all, but a significant reduction in calories on certain days. One of the first things you should know about intermittent fasting is that consistency is important. You are going to be eating on a schedule and finding the right schedule for you is what is going to be your key to success.

Fasting Methods

16/8 Method: This is one of the most popular methods of fasting because it is so schedule based, meaning there are no surprises. This gives you the freedom to control when you eat based on your daily life. The 16 is the number of hours you are going to be fasting, which can also be lowered to 12 or 14 hours if that fits into your life better. Then your eating period will be between 8 and 10 hours each day. This might seem daunting, but it really just means that you are skipping an entire meal. Many people choose to begin their fast around 7 or 8 p.m. and then do not eat until 11 or noon the next day, which means they are fasting for the recommended 16 hours. Of course, it isn't as bad as it sounds since they are also sleeping during this time too, so what it really comes down to is eating dinner and then not eating again the next day around lunch, so you are just skipping breakfast.

You will be doing this every day, so finding the hours that work for you are important. If you work third shift, then switching your eating period around to fit into your schedule is important. Also, if you find yourself being run down and sluggish, then tweak your fasting hours until you find a healthy balance. Granted, there is going to be some adjustment, because, chances are, your body is not accustomed to skipping entire meals. However, this should go away after a couple of weeks, and if it doesn't then try starting your fasting period earlier in the day allowing you to eat earlier the next, or alter it however you need to feel healthy and happy.

5:2 Method: This is another popular way to fast, because there is no true fasting involved, but instead a strict and drastic reduction of calories for two days each week. So, for five days a week, you are going to eat your normal 1.600 to 2,000 calories and exercising like normal. The on two nonconsecutive days a week you are going to restrict your caloric intake to between 500 and 600 calories. When doing this pay close attention the number of calories in beverages as well, many people make the mistake of only counting calories in what they eat. Remember, that beverages contain calories too, especially if you are drinking things from coffee shops, as these have a tendency to have high amounts of sugar.

Eat-Stop-Eat Method: This method requires the longest fasting period and therefore is not right for everyone. For five days out of the week you are going to be eating normally, again, between 1,600 and 2,000 calories and then you are going to fast for two 24 hour periods. That means no food will be consumed at all for two days each week, these should not be consecutive days. Even though this seems like a long time to go without eating, your body can adjust to this and a lot of people prefer this method because they can schedule their fasting days during the week on days that they know are rather slow. If this is the method you choose, you should also know that on fasting days it is important to not push yourself too hard when exercising. What you do drink on fasting days should not contain sugar, many people stick with water, tea, and black coffee. Some people also like to drink bone broth on these days too, but what you drink is completely up to you.

Crescendo Method: This is usually an introduction to fasting, it is how many people begin their fasting journey. This is a less intense form of intermittent fasting and is a great way for you to see how it works to ease your fears and become familiarized with a fasting schedule. This method involves normally for 4 or 5 days a week and then restricting your eating period to between 8 or 10 hours for two or three nonconsecutive days. Very similar to the 16/8 method, but instead of doing this every day, you only do it a couple days each week. Again, this is a great way to introduce your mind and body to the world of intermittent fasting. You can also choose which days and how many hours your fasting will be, giving you the control to fit into your life as comfortably as possible.

These are the safest ways for women to fast because they do not upset the hormonal balance of the body. Intermittent fasting not done properly can trick the body into going into what is known as starvation mode. This happens when the body thinks it needs to hold onto fat longer because it doesn't know when it will have a chance to consume food for fuel again. This can lead to burning muscle for fuel as well as upsetting the hormonal balance, leading to even more issues. However, intermittent fasting done properly can be safe and incredibly beneficial.

Not only does intermittent fasting help you lose weight, but it also improves mental clarity and allows you to simplify your life in a way that diets do not. Think about how much time you spend worrying about or eating food, and then imagine what other things you could be doing if this were not the case. This is one the major benefits of intermittent fasting, there are no surprises and you are able to take complete control of when you eat.

Like many people you are probably assuming that you are going to overdo it on calories when you do start your eating period. Yes, that might be the case in the beginning because your body is going through an adjustment, but that is generally not the case after a few days. Think of it like this, you eat dinner around 7 p.m. and then you skip breakfast the next day. You are definitely going to be hungry around lunchtime, as is natural, and your lunch can be a large, healthy meal that is about 750 calories, similar to your dinner, both of which are probably going to a bit larger than if you were not skipping breakfast. Then, it doesn't stop there, you are still allotted the standard amount of calories during the 8 to 10 hour eating period which means you still have 300 or 500 calories to spend on dessert or a sugary beverage. You are depriving yourself of anything and you saved yourself between 500 to 700 calories just by skipping breakfast.

When you break it down like that, it doesn't seem nearly as scary. Then if you decide to the 5:2 method, you are not going to long without eating at all, but instead paying very close attention to what you do eat on your restricting days. The same concept still applies, stick to a schedule and pay careful, close attention to all calories consumed. One of the most common ways people do this is by eating whole, clean foods only on those days and not consuming any empty calories at all. You'd be surprised how many vegetables you can eat before you reach 300 calories. This prevents you from feeling hungry for very long or at all throughout the day.

No matter what method you choose, it is important to stick to a strict schedule. This is how you are going to be eating from now on. Getting a calendar and marking your fasting or restricting days helps because you can see it in front of you. Make sure these days are nonconsecutive and make them the same every week. You have a life, so take all of your obligations into consideration when you are deciding which days to restrict or fast, or what time your fasting period will begin and end.

Part of your life might and definitely should include exercising, maybe you are a regular at a Pilates class, or you are training for a marathon. Intermittent fasting can accommodate this aspect of your life too. You just need to know how to work your exercise routines into your fasting schedule or vice versa. If you decide on the Eat-stop-eat method or 5:2 method, there are going to be days when you consume nearly no calories or are restricting, and to avoid light headedness and fatigue, use those days for either relaxation or to do light exercising such as yoga or light jogging. Intermittent fasting is not meant to feel like torture or to make you feel worse. So, keep that in mind when you are making your schedule, it will help you succeed in the long run.

It doesn't matter what you eat during your eating period as long you stay within the healthy amount of calories. Yet, it is no surprise that the healthier you do eat, the better your results are going to be. So, if you are already a healthy eater, just keep that diet up. If you are not a very healthy eater, consider making some small changes to your diet, it will lead to better results. One of the best things about intermittent fasting is that you will see results fast and it will improve your overall discipline as you become familiar with your new eating schedule. Nothing serves as better motivation than results, so without even trying many people find that they want to improve their diet because they want to see even more results.

Now you understand the basics and you have probably already made a decision about which method or methods you are going to try. That's great, you should be picky about which one is right for you, as no people are the same and intermittent fasting allows you to control your eating schedule. Despite which method you choose, you should definitely know that there is going to be an adjustment period for both your mind and body. Lifestyle changes are not always easy and they do require self-discipline. Of course, this comes more naturally to some than others, however, everyone is capable of making a change. The more prepared you are for what is to come, the more likely you are to stick with it and succeed.

The adjustment process is when your body is adapting to the new eating schedule you have put it on. It is uncomfortable, you are going to feel rundown, frustrated, irritable, and hungry in the beginning. These symptoms do not last very long, your body is capable of adapting rather quickly, as you'll see. This is one of the most crucial parts of intermittent fasting – listening to your body. If you get passed what you think is the adjustment period and you still not feel well, it is time to take a look at your schedule and figure out what changes need to be made to make you feel better. There are many ways to go about this, you can either shorten your fasting period or switch the times, or just move your fasting or restricting days to different days of the week. For some people, they prefer their fasting days to be weekdays so they can focus on work, have a light workout and then relax. Other people like to have their restriction days be Fridays or Saturdays because they know those are days off work and they can spend their time just relaxing. This is a personal choice and listening to your body is the best way to make these decisions.

Now you're probably worried about how you can intermittent fast and have any semblance of a normal social life. That is a common fear for many people when they begin intermittent fasting. No matter which method, there are times of restricting and fasting, both of which can throw a wrench into one's personal lives. There is no quick solution to this, but there are ways to make it happen. Your lifestyle changed the moment you began intermittent fasting, and that includes your social life. Granted, intermittent fasting is going to impact all aspects of your life, but there are ways to minimize the negative and make sure you are not miserable. This cannot be stressed enough, intermittent fasting does not and should not make you more stressed or cause you to feel unhappy. The opposite is true, you should feel energized, more alert, focused, and able to live a more simplified life.

Figuring out how to have a normal social and work life while intermittent fasting can be tricky because just as intermittent fasting is not one-size-fits-all, neither is the solution. Everyone is different and so are their lives and schedules. Planning is the most important part of making sure you can indeed have it all. The more prepared you are, the more likely you are to have a more seamless transition, which only helps you succeed. As you continue on your intermittent fasting journey, don' t be afraid to make a detailed schedule, use your phone or even get a hard copy planner if that is what helps you. There are many different options and with intermittent fasting, there are many different options and schedules available to you. Also, don't be afraid of failing. Sometimes it takes some trial and error before you find out what works for you. So until you do find that balance, don' t be too hard on yourself and learn to celebrate the small steps. It is often these small steps that lead to big changes because they help you find what ultimately will work for you.

Chapter 2: Understand Your Priorities

Intermittent fasting is a schedule, you are now on a different eating schedule than you were before. You are either going days with restricting calories or fasting, or have a set eating period that you must adhere to in order to reap the benefits and be successful. That being said, it can also seem like in order to stick to this schedule you are going to make a lot of sacrifices when it comes to your social life. Yes, you might have make some changes, but if done properly, you won't have to completely miss out on anything.

One of the first things you need to do is to make a list of everything goes on your life in an average week. This might seem crazy, but chances are you don't know how busy you are until you see it in front of you in black and white. Just think about all those days that you feel as though you are being pulled in many different directions, work, family obligations, making time for friends, trying to find time to take a relaxing bath, and then maybe you need to take your dog for a walk. Life is hard because there are so many hours in a day and so many days in a week.

Intermittent fasting is just going to add another schedule into your life that already has scheduled events and routines. So, to make things as easy as possible make that list, include absolutely everything on there that you do, including the family functions, times you generally hang out with friends, the times you actually can sneak away for some personal time. Include everything, as this the list that is going to help you make intermittent fasting work for how you live.

Once your list is complete, take a close look at everything you have included. There are some things that are non-negotiable as far as higher priorities, such as work. However, this is a list of your daily life and how intermittent fasting is going to impact that. Fortunately, work can be done without eating since your time is already occupied with working.

However, let's assume that you have a standing hangout with friends that starts at 7 every Friday, and this is important to you. It is so important in fact that you don't want to have to abstain from food while all your friends are happily eating around you. That's absolutely okay, you are making this an important priority in your life, something that makes you happy. So, either do not schedule as one of your fasting days or make the effort and decision to start your fasting period later at night and make it last later into the following day. Just remember, that if you do that, you cannot change it back on the days that you do not meet with friends. This might mean that you are going to be eating a later lunch and dinner, but in the grand scheme of things, you are not going to be missing out on anything.

Furthermore, when you are looking at your list, let's say that you also have a work obligation that takes place late on a weeknight a couple of times a month. Your colleagues might meet late for drinks, well into your fasting period. This is going to be one of the more difficult and uncomfortable times because you are going to have to abstain. In this sense, you are making your intermittent fasting lifestyle your priority. When this happens, get creative when you are out. Don't skip going all together, instead order a soda water with lime or hot tea and continue on as usual.

Yes, this is a different type of lifestyle than you were living before, but you knew changes were going to be made when you began your journey. When you have the list of things that are important to you in front of you, it is easier to schedule your fasting period or days around what makes you feel sane and happy. You work hard and intermittent fasting is not meant to take everything away from you. No, it just might take some creative rescheduling to make it work.

One of the most common issues someone has when they begin intermittent fasting is the situation that was previously described. So, this is the cold, hard, truth – you are going to go out and fast. Try not to make it a habit until you adapt to your new eating schedule but do accept that fact. Learn to find little tricks or hacks, that make doing this easier for you. Some people like to drink a lot of water to make themselves feel full, which is a very option. Others like to sip on tea or coffee throughout the night. In the beginning, this might feel like torture, as a matter of fact, you might find yourself leaving early. However, the longer you intermittent fast, the easier situations like these will become.

The reason this happens is that you are retraining the way your brain thinks about food. Eating becomes a scheduled way to consume food for fuel and not something that is done for boredom or social reasons. This takes some time to get used to, but it will happen and once it does, you'll be much more comfortable in these types of situations. Just don't put too much pressure on yourself in the beginning, of course, try not to break your fast, but if you do, simply treat it as a learning opportunity and move on the next day.

However, if this type of thing keeps happening, it might actually be a priority of yours. So it might be time to go back your schedule and make the necessary alterations to your fasting schedule to fit this particular routine social event into your eating period. There is nothing wrong with doing this, that is the whole of point of intermittent fasting. You get to choose when you eat and when you fast based on your specific schedule and needs.

Know the Difference Between a Priority and a Simple Want

Intermittent fasting is not something that you can start and then stop whenever you want. You need to be ready to make a complete lifestyle change, which takes time to make sure you will lose or maintain a healthy weight. Makings the list of everything you do during the week is meant to help you sort through what your needs and wants are. You might not always get what you want, but intermittent fasting can definitely be made to make sure your needs are adequately met.

This means that when you look at that list, you are going to have to think about what your habits are. More often than not, there is more than you think that you don't actually need, therefore are not considered priorities so you do not need to take these into consideration when making your fasting schedule. A great example of this would be a midnight snack or drinks after 10 p.m. both of these are examples of wants, but not necessarily priorities. Alcohol is one of those things that some intermittent fasters would say is never allowed, but others say it can be as long as the calories are deducted properly. However, there is no reason for you to drink after the fasting period begins. This is not something that is a priority and part of the lifestyle change. Therefore, it is another example of when the intermittent fasting lifestyle is actually the priority. The same goes for that midnight snack you have come to depend on. Sure, you like it, but you do not need it and your fasting schedule does not need to incorporate it.

On the other hand. If you are training for a marathon or just like a heavy workout throughout the week, then this would be a priority. Finding out how your body reacts to a workout and food consumption is the best way to handle this, for instance, maybe you deal better eating a large breakfast and then working out, if that is the case, begin your fasting period earlier in the day so your eating period begins earlier the next morning before your workout. Everyone is different in this regard so it could take some time and trial and error before you figure out how to make both of this work, but you will figure out what is the most important to you.

The end goal is to find a balance between what you have given up in order to stick to an intermittent fasting schedule, and how to substitute other things or times to make up for that loss. So, let's say that you can no longer have that early brunch on

Sundays that you normally do because of your fasting period. Come to terms with that or ask if you can switch the time to an hour or two later. Or just tell the people that you're with that you are fasting on that day because it fits into your schedule best and that you will still be there, but a little bit later so that you don't have to be present while others eat in front of you. This temptation will continue, but time and experience will make it much easier for you to cope with. Many people who are intermittent fasters have found that once their bodies adapt to their new way of eating, situations such as these, barely bother them anymore.

Some people are going to find that they adjust faster than others and one of the best things do is not to compare yourself to others. Everyone is going to react and adjust in different ways and that's okay. If you need to stick with the social events and obligations that only fit into your eating periods at the beginning that just do that. There is nothing wrong with taking your time while you figure out what your priorities are making sure to fit them into your busy day to day life.

Intermittent fasting is going to be a priority of its own, as you can see, sometimes that is what is going to take precedence over other things. That's the nature of a lifestyle change – change. You wouldn't be reading this or wanting to take the leap into intermittent fasting if there wasn't a reason, whether it is to lose weight, gain energy, or just to simplify your life. That means that you are making intermittent fasting a priority right there. It is important to you.

When you start to make the changes you'll also see how your body begins to handle everything and this can also help you determine what your priorities truly are. For instance, it might not be that hard to go out with friends right after your fasting period began because you ate at home and you just simply aren't hungry so it isn't difficult to not eat. Other times you will find that you are eating for boredom and that you aren't really hungry and intermittent fasting teaches you rather quickly to listen to your body so you can interpret the signals its sending you. You might be surprised how often you eat not because you are actually hungry, but just because there is nothing else to do.

Intermittent fasting also allows for you to snack if you are more a grazer type eater, rather than two larger meals a day. There's a simple solution to this, just keep doing it, but make sure you keep the caloric intake at a healthy limit and begin fasting at your normal time. Again, there is no wrong or right way to do this, it is simply part of the process, finding what works best for you.

One of the last things that you might to be important when you are considering your priorities is whether or not you want to tell your friends. Intermittent fasting is still rather controversial simply because people are not educated about it and you'll quickly find that nearly everyone has an opinion about it. Sometimes these opinions are going to be negative and again, negativity is not going to set you on the path to success. As a matter of fact, it can be one of the main reasons someone decides to stop intermittent fasting altogether. If you are worried about that, do what many other people do and just say that you just ate or that you are trying to eat at home to save money. The choice of how you handle this is up to you. Just know that this is a common occurrence and the more prepared you are for every situation, this included, is going to help you.

Chapter 3: You Can Go Out and Fast

Welcome to one of the biggest challenges of intermittent fasting, when you have no choice but to go to a dinner or a hangout with friends during your fasting period. This is one of the most difficult parts of the transition to intermittent fasting because it is something that our brain has not been introduced to. You have probably been going out with friends on a regular basis for a long time and these social gatherings generally also contain food.

There is no simple solution to this, it's going to be difficult, especially in the beginning. No matter how much you plan, there is going to be a time when there is an obligation that happens to fall on a fasting day or during a fasting period. It's something that you simply can't avoid. When you find yourself in this situation, and you will, how you handle it will be the determining factor in how successful you are going to be.

First, if you are doing the 16/8 or the Crescendo method you know exactly when your fasting period starts. Before your social engagement that you know will be full of food related temptations, eat a large meal right before the end of your eating period. You can make this a more carbohydrate heavy meal or choose other foods that will keep you full longer. This way when you do go out, you know it is your brain telling you to eat because you should, not your body telling you to eat because you're hungry. This is what it means to reset your brain. You have spent so much of your life training your brain to associate food with different situations that actually have very little to do with real hunger. Now you are faced with the difficult task of trying to change that.

This change is not going to happen overnight, but again, it will get easier with time and experience. A lot of intermittent fasters know the importance of drinking water, it keeps you hydrated and in times of temptation can also help make you feel full. Most of the time situations like these take good old fashioned discipline and the ability to just abstain. You know you are going to be able to eat soon and eat what you want, it just won't happen right then. Telling yourself that might be a helpful mantra to help you get through the difficult times when eating is just not an option because intermittent fasting is the priority.

Since there is no easy solution to this, acceptance is the easiest solution. You know that life is hectic and that even the most scheduled plans can somehow get changed or ruined at the last minute. Intermittent fasting is no exception, you are now on a different eating schedule, one that might begin or end earlier than you are normally customary with. On one hand, you do know when you are going to able to eat, but on the other, you are surrounded by food. Every intermittent faster has been there and knows they will be again the future. It's inevitable really.

Part of intermittent fasting is listening to your body and breaking the habit of eating simply because you are in the position to do so. Eating when you are hungry and intermittent fasting are both examples of mindful eating. You are feeding your body during the set times that you have chosen, so rationally you know you aren't starving. However, this does not help with reducing or eliminating temptation. Intermittent fasting does help teach you to listen to your body, but you are also attempting to undo years of unmindful eating. Some people might not even know when they're full in the beginning and often overdo it when their eating period begins. That's when counting general calories helps you because in the beginning, you might be able to depend on your brain, but you can depend on the actual caloric number to show yourself that you are not really hungry, you have been consuming enough calories for your body.

The more comfortable and confident you are about being able to tell yourself that you are full or that you will be able to eat the soon, the easier situations like this are going to be. When you first begin intermittent fasting, the more difficult it is going to be to say no to temptations like office birthday parties or unplanned outings that involve food. So, should you find yourself unable to abstain completely, do not go overboard and simply start back the next day. Do not make a habit of this but do learn to forgive yourself if you occasionally break your fast early or eat a little something on fasting days. The longer you intermittent fast, the easier it will be to say no to these things.

Before you go out, have a positive attitude and do not assume that you are going to break your fast. Instead, prepare yourself mentally by figuring out what you are going to tell people about why you are not eating or drinking. You can say that you are only eating at home or be honest and just say that you stop eating at 7 p.m. for health reasons. Many people prefer to tell people that as soon as they get to whatever event it is that they're going to so that they can spend their time talking to others, which goes a long way in taking the mind off of food.

Taking food out of the equation during social situations can be challenging, but it can also be a learning experience. Take that time to really have conversations with others, most people are surprised at how quickly time flies when they are keeping focused on other things. A great example of this is having fun, if you are out with friends for a party of some kind, there are going to be other opportunities to do things other than eating, some of these are going to be more obvious than others. If karaoke is going on, take advantage and get up there and sing. Sometimes it is not going to be that easy, but you can always find the other people who are already done eating and join them for a conversation. The good news is, dinners do not last forever, so there is an end in sight. It's okay to constantly remind yourself of that if you find yourself in a situation when it is hard to refrain.

Put yourself first, you might be out with friends, but you also don't need to be miserable. A little bit of planning for this can go a long way. Finding out who is planning whatever the event maybe and asking for a schedule could help you seek out alternatives such as sitting at the bar and drinking a soda water. Sometimes all it takes is having one person that will support you to make all the difference, even they don't now the whole truth and just assume you're on a diet, having someone in your corner just makes it easier. If you think that is what you need, then absolutely do it. Some intermittent fasters also have a friend that sends them texts or is there for them to call before or after times of temptation to talk, knowing others are in the same boat as you can also be helpful.

Learning to have fun without food is a challenge, but you're capable of doing it, as so many others have too. Just like the different methods of intermittent fasting, there are many different tactics to having fun while going out and fasting. Some events are going to be easier than others, such as a baby shower is going to be an easier situation because there are people mingling around, games to be played, and just general conversation. On the other hand, a sit down work dinner is going to be more difficult because the entire occasion is about food. Events like this, while yes, they are based on food, it also means that the food portion of the evening will come to an end at some point and then conversation will be the focus and until that happens, finding yourself drinking more water than usual is most definitely a common coping mechanism and something you should not feel bad about.

In the beginning, you might yourself dreading going out because you feel as though any social event is going to be like this. However, the nature of scheduled eating and planned social life typically means that won't be a problem. You have worked hard making your fasting schedule and finding the method that works for you, so more than likely, you will be more naturally committed to this lifestyle than you thought. Humans have a tendency to not want to ruin or sabotage something they've worked hard for. Allow that work in your favor, you are allowed to be proud of what you have worked towards and telling people that you are going to go out and not eat, but still have a great time is something you have definitely earned. This is also going to be something that continuously comes up when you are an intermittent faster, so the better you get at, the easier.

It's hard not to be too hard on yourself, there's a reason that people say, "you are your own worst critic." Sometimes we stand in our way and beat ourselves up too much if we fail. Intermittent fasting is a journey, one that you are going to make mistakes during, learning from those mistakes and making changes so it doesn't happen again is part of the process. So instead of being afraid of it, learn to embrace change and the minor failings that are inevitable. There is no one else in the world with a body and brain just like yours. Remember, you are taking something and making it fit for you specifically, there is no direct guide book for this. You are basically making it up as you go along. It's only natural to make mistakes, but you also need to learn to celebrate the things you do right. Having a positive attitude in general, both at home and while going out is only going to help you.

Even though there is no simple solution for going out and fasting, you can and will still find your own way. Once you start to see results and evaluate your priorities, there will be very little to hold you back. Your outlook on life is going to change the longer you continue to intermittent fast because you start to understand what your body is capable of. You will start to view food in a different way as well, no longer as a means to solve boredom or as a social event, but as what it is, a source of energy for your body. This is a natural progression and byproduct of intermittent fasting. This new outlook is also one of the biggest motivators for wanting to stay on track when you do go out, you will start to see that going out and hanging out with friends does not need to revolve around food.

When you combine everything you've learned and accomplished during your first couple of weeks of intermittent fasting things will start to come together in a way that makes more sense to you. Everything you've read will now be something you understand in terms of practice and not just words on a page. Being shy about changing your schedule or altering your eating habits will come much more naturally. All of this is what contributes to your confidence and your ability to stay committed to the lifestyle change you made. Even though the start is a bit rocky, you'll quickly see that it does get easier. Your life will start to become more simplified because food will no longer be a source of stress. Going out will take on a new meaning to you. Eating will become something that is used for energy and your life will have a more simplified tone.

Chapter 4: Planning Ahead, Learning How to Fast and Be Happy

There are so many things in life that simply can't be planned, but when you eat shouldn't be one of them. Knowing when and what you are going to eat saves you time, increases the chances of making healthy choices, and simplifies your life. Intermittent fasting has many different methods to choose from with different schedules that fit into your life. Having different options in terms of schedules and when your eating period begins and ends gives you more time to spend doing other things.

Taking this a step further and meal planning and prepping is one of the easiest ways to stick to intermittent fasting. All of the guessing is removed from what you eat, along with the stress of what comes with it. When you made your list of priorities, you figured out your eating schedule based on what is important to you. So, you already know when you are going to be eating, regardless of which method you chose.

Each intermittent fasting method, although similar, is still a little different so meal planning and prepping for each is going to be different. Remember that based on which method you choose; your grocery list is going to reflect this. If you are on the 16/8 method then more than likely, you are skipping breakfast, so when you grocery shop, there is no reason to get breakfast foods. Your focus can be on lunch and dinner ingredients which are often interchangeable and can be mixed in different ways. This can also save you money too since there are many items that you won't be eating anymore.

The same can be said for the 5:2 method because you are going to be skipping meals two or three days a week. It's important to take that into consideration when you are grocery shopping as well. Another thing to remember is that you are in control of your eating schedule and how you eat. If your body reacts better to eating two big meals, then focus on purchasing items that you can make into two larger meals. If grazing suits you better, then purchase items that you can pack with you to take to work and out with you to eat during your eating period. You'll learn what works best for you and be able to cater to that while grocery shopping.

If you want to take all the guessing out of eating, meal prepping is right for you. Many intermittent fasters do this is as it really does a lot to simplify their lives. You can do this by making a weekly plan of what you are going to eat for each meal and then purchasing the necessary ingredients. However, it doesn't stop there. You are also going to prep the meals so you can easily throw your lunch into your bag or toss some ingredients into a crockpot. However, you decide to do it is up to you.

How to Meal Prep

This might be your first time meal prepping, so it's important to educate yourself on how it works.

First, you are going to pick a day in which you are going to prep all your meals for the week. Some intermittent fasters choose to do this on a day when they are fasting for 24 hours if they are doing the eat-stop-eat method because it is an easy way to spend their time and occupy themselves. Others find that meal prepping on these days increases their temptation to eat too much, so listen to your body and do what's right for you.

Just like making your list of priorities, it helps to have your food list set out in front of you in black and white as a reference. You know what days are busiest and at what times you like to indulge in some more sugar heavy desserts. Having it written out in front of you gives you the visual you need to make sure you aren't missing anything. Be sure to include beverages as well, since some people would rather forgo dessert in favor of a mocha or sugary beverage that takes up those allotted calories.

Once you have all the meals planned out and are happy with what you have, you are going to simply prep the meals just as though you were going to be cooking dinner or taking your lunch with you. Many people like to buy enough Tupperware to fill their fridge with their prepped meals, while others like to use one large container and separate the portions. However you decide to do it is fine, it's your choice. Next, you are going to just assemble everything in individual portions so you can quickly put together a healthy lunch, whether it be making a stacked salad in a jar or cooking a protein and then freezing it so it can be quickly warmed up at the office. This is personal preference; your goal is just to make your chosen meals more convenient and to take the guessing out of meal preparation.

When meal prepping it is also important to remember that, depending on which method of intermittent fasting you practice, there might be whole days in which you go without eating. So, you find that your salads or greens are wilting quickly or things just don't taste as fresh, you might want to reconsider how you prep and only do it for a couple of days at a time. Many intermittent fasters prefer to do it this way because it lets them easily switch up their meal plans if they find themselves craving something specific.

Meal prepping can go as far as cooking everything for the week and then placing it in the freezer and warming up meals. Or it can be simply creating portions and then cooking them each night. There is no right or wrong to do this, however, it fits into your schedule and life is the right way. Meal prepping and planning lets you make the right food choices to fuel your body. As you progress with intermittent fasting you might find that you prefer certain foods for a specific reason, like eating heavier before exercising. Meal prepping makes this easier because you can have that larger portion already measured out and ready to go. On the other hand, if you are someone who prefers to eat smaller meals throughout the day, having smaller portions all ready to go makes it a lot easier too.

One of the major benefits of meal planning and prepping is that you are cooking at home and you are in complete control of what goes into the meals you eat. That means you are able to quickly look up the calorie count of everything you eat to make sure you are within the healthy limits and not overdoing it. This is very important for 5:2 fasters as well as anyone who is just beginning intermittent fasting since it is a natural desire to want to eat more when first skipping meals. When your portions are already made for you and all you have to do is throw the ingredients in a microwave, crockpot, skillet, or oven, after a long day at work. That's what you are going to do. If you eat your prepped meal and find that you are still hungry, wait half an hour and then see how you feel. Your body is adjusting and sometimes it takes the brain a little while to catch up to the fact that your body is indeed full.

Some people would rather not meal prep at all, instead, they would rather lightly meal plan or just stick to what they know and switch it up every day. For those who take joy in cooking meals and choosing what sounds good to them on any particular day, intermittent fasting will still work just as well.

Intermittent fasting is just changing when you eat, so if cooking is a passion, all you have to do is know when to do it. There is no reason for you to stop doing something you enjoy.

General Planning

As mentioned before, you are going to find yourself in a situation in which you are going to have to alter your schedule. Planning ahead is still going to help you though. Looking at your weekly schedule of plans means that you know what you are going to do and when. If you have a party planned on a Saturday night that begins at 5 p.m. which is the same time you have your last big meal of the night, it would help you to eat earlier. You can still how up on time and full by simply changing your dinner time. There is no reason to do this every Saturday, but sometimes situations like this arise and small changes can make all the difference.

Another thing to consider when planning is what you crave and when. As most women know, there are certain times of the month in which less attention is paid to maintaining a healthy diet. Planning for these days beforehand is a great way to stay on track and still enjoy the cravings you normally have. Many sources on intermittent fasting leave out information about how to fast during menstruation, but it can be done. Granted, it is going much more difficult for those who are practicing the eat-stop-eat method, because they might be faced with cravings on a fasting day. To help with this, some people drink more coffee, while others find a tea and use a sugar substitute to help satisfy a craving without breaking their fast. Of course, there are also healthier alternatives to sweet foods in general, such as switching to dark chocolate, or frozen yogurt. Whatever your specific cravings are, take to doing some research to find healthier versions so you can make that time easier on yourself.

It's also a good idea to plan for vacations too. Some intermittent fasters simply quit for a vacation because it is important to them to try new and different foods while they are travelling. That's okay if it is simply for a vacation because they do not happen often. Just be sure to not overindulge and then to go right back to intermittent fasting when you return. If your vacation is going to be long, you might want to still choose to limit your calories or to still choose a day to fast for a full 24 hours. Again, this is personal preference, listening to your body and focusing on how you feel is the key to finding that balance. However, if travel is a part of your regular life, that is a different case and intermittent fasting should be a priority.

As you can see, the secret to successfully intermittent fasting is consistency and scheduling. Before you start it might seem downright terrifying, the thought of skipping meals every day or not eating at all for two days every week. However, once you start your chosen method, your mind and body will both adjust and it will come much more naturally than it did when you first started. You will find yourself being able to go out into social situations and not worry about eating. Intermittent fasting and your new eating schedule will quickly be your normal eating habits. When this happens, you'll be pleased to see that what was challenging, in the beginning, is just no longer an issue. Intermittent fasting has a tendency to increase self-discipline in all parts of your life without you even realizing it. Consider it one of the many benefits of intermittent fasting.

As you continue your fasting journey, you will see many changes happening to your body. You will have increased mental alertness, less body fat, and more energy. All of these serve as natural motivators to want to continue. So even if it feels difficult in the beginning, the results happen relatively quickly and you will be able to see all of your hard work paying off. Know what your reasons were for starting intermittent fasting were in the first place, whether it be to lose weight or simplify your life, you will be able to reap the many benefits that come with the change in lifestyle.

Chapter 5: Tips for Going Out or Hanging Out While Fasting

You already know that there are going to be times when you are not eating, but still, have to go out and be surrounded by both food and other people eating. This is not an easy situation to be in for anyone, but it is even more difficult for those who are just starting to intermittent fast. Even though these situations cannot be avoided altogether there are some things that can be done to make life a little easier for you when they do. As you probably already know, the more prepared you are, the more likely you are to succeed. Even though the way you hangout and approach your social life is going to be different than it was before, you are still capable of having both – intermittent fasting and a social life.

Tips

Buddy System – There are many ways to go about finding someone to help you when you need it. Intermittent fasting means making a lot of changes and temptations will arise. Sometimes having someone to text or call makes it a lot easier to deal with those times. One thing you can do is to go to someone you are close to and really trust. Keep in mind that a lot of people do not fully understand what intermittent fasting entails so be prepared to explain it. If you make it clear to someone that cares for you that is important to you to make this switch, then they will be more likely to help you. This means that even if someone is not an intermittent faster, they can still act as a support system.

Another popular way of finding someone to help you stay on track is to find someone who is going through the same things you are – another beginner intermittent faster. This can be done pretty easily by joining a group or forum online and asking if anyone wants an intermittent fasting buddy. Think of it as a new way to make a friend and to both receive and give support when needed. Just talking about challenges and successes with someone who understands can serve as a great reason to stay on track because it just simply helps to not feel alone.

Bring Food – You might be able to bring your own food and beverages into a restaurant, but that doesn't you can't take them to a friend's house. This is, of course, a case-by-case basis, but take some bone broth with you if you know you are going to an event that is based on food. This way you are still consuming something, it will go a long way into making you feel more comfortable too. Some intermittent fasters even go as far as to putting the broth they brought with them into their friend's bowls so it doesn't look like they brought their own food alternative at all. Many people only do this in the beginning, before they get more comfortable, but doing what you can to make you feel better and more comfortable is important.

Don't be Shy – If it is a day in which you are restricting your calories, but find yourself out with friends, don't be shy about asking the exact calorie amount in the food. You need to be careful about what you order and sometimes it is going to take some time to find out what is acceptable. Ask questions, pay attention to the ala carte menu and the sides. Sometimes making a small entrée out of two sides is the best way to create a low-calorie meal from a menu that doesn't offer low calorie options. Another option is to choose a low-calorie meal and then only eating half of it since most low-calorie meals are still around 500 calories which is the limit for the 5:2 method. By only eating half of it, you have a better idea of how many calories you are actually consuming, which is better than not having any clue at all.

Creative Drink Orders – Many people have a favorite coffee shop and beverage to go along with it. Just as many people might be shocked to find out how many calories and sugar are in that beverage as well. This when it is time to get creative and do some research. If you love frozen coffee drinks, a good alternative is get an iced coffee blended, you might get a strange look, but it is just black coffee and ice, but in that blended way you enjoy so much. If you normally get a caramel or vanilla drink, ask for what syrups they offer that are sugar-free and make that switch. You can even substitute almond or soy milk too if your chosen drinks contains heavy cream. It might not be the exact same, but you can find something that still tastes good and doesn't take up so much of your caloric intake. This also means that you can still drink something fun when visiting friends at a coffee shop.

Water – This should go without saying, but drink water. Staying hydrated is important and it is crucial when you are going longer periods without eating. If you start to feel hungry drink some water, your eating period will begin, but before it does drinking water might help to curb your appetite. Switch it up, drink hot water in the morning with a splash of lemon juice or if you normally drink hot water, make yourself a giant glass of ice water. You can even switch to sparkling or mineral water too if you choose. However, stay away from flavored waters from the store since they are often full of sugars or sugar substitutes. It's better to keep it simple and to know what it is you are drinking.

Vitamins – Even though you are still eating a healthy diet and consuming a normal amount of calories, it is still a good idea to take a multivitamin or some supplements. You don't have to stock your cabinets with an array of different supplements, but it is a good idea to take a multivitamin. This will help you increase your energy and boost your metabolism. Some people do choose to take different supplements, especially on days when they are fasting for a full 24 hours because it can help with increasing energy and preventing sluggishness and fatigue. Making a trip to a local vitamin shop is a great place to start if you know very little about supplements, the people who work there can help you find exactly what you're looking for with no judgment.

Bring Your Meals – Sometimes it not going out when you are in a fasting period that is the challenge but going out during an eating period that is. Some people who meal plan or prep do not like to deviate from the meals they have planned if you are one of these people then be prepared to get creative and don't be shy. If you are going to a restaurant, you are probably not going to be able to bring in your own food. However, not all states are the same, and honestly, some restaurants just don't care. It doesn't hurt to call ahead and ask if you are told no, eat your meal as close as you can to the time before you leave so you are still full. If you are going to a friend's house or even a picnic, bring your own food, your friends probably won't have an issue with it, and if they do, just explain that you are meal prepping and consistency is important.

Be adventurous - Try to be the one who organizes events with your friends when you can and find places that offer different tea or coffee choices. This might seem strange, but sometimes just the act of introducing a new flavor to your palette will be enough to satisfy the urge to eat with friends. Try out different types of foods, your friends can try something new in terms of the food menu and you can find a new type of tea you haven't had before.

Fruit water - If you are going to be hanging out a friend's house for a cookout, but you know it happens on one of your fasting days, bring some cold, refreshing fruit water with you. Granted, those around you might be drinking beer or cocktails and eating burgers or hotdogs, but you are committed to a lifestyle change, so you already knew that there were going some things that you are going to have to give up. In general, citrus fruits are not high in sugar and you will be able to enjoy something that is both healthy and flavorful. This is something that you do not make a habit off because those calories will add up, but for times when you know you will be hanging out with friends in a time like that, this is a great alternative.

Be Honest – Depending on who your friends are and what kind of personality you have, just telling everyone of your lifestyle change might be the best option. If you think your friends will react positively, or if you know you can handle criticism and continue with intermittent fasting, then this can go a long way in helping you stay on track. The more support you feel like you have the more likely you are to keep on the right path. Even if your friends do not intermittent fast themselves, they are still in a position to help you. So, if this an option for you, take it, you never know when there will be people there to help you.

After you have progressed to the point of both your mind and body accepting your new eating schedule, everything else has a tendency to fall into place. Just let things happen at a normal pace and try not to push yourself too hard. Patience is important when making a lifestyle change, your life is not supposed to revolve around your eating schedule, but rather your eating schedule should fit into your life. Finding that balance might take some time and until you get there, remember that this is a journey and that there are going to be some obstacles involved.

One of these main obstacles is finding a way to both intermittent fast and maintain your social life. If you need to skip somethings in the beginning, then do so, but don't continue that habit. You know what your priorities are and a healthy social life is part of that. Granted, there are going to be some changes, but you will not need to sacrifice your social life altogether. Intermittent fasting does not mean barricading yourself in your home when you aren't working. Even if that does like an appealing option in the beginning, with some experience and patience, this feeling will fade and you will find yourself with more energy and a desire to want that active social life you had before.

No matter what stage you're in of intermittent fasting, remember that's it's still important to have fun. This is your life, you are simply taking control of when and how you eat. Yes, there will be other repercussions to that decision, but that also means that you have the control to make sure you aren't missing out anything too. Whether it be finding a fasting buddy or meal prepping, there are many different ways to make this lifestyle transition easier for you. Some of the time you are going to feel great about your choice, and other times you are going to wonder what on Earth you have gotten yourself into. That is a natural feeling, nearly everyone who makes a lifestyle change has this feeling. What you do about it is what is going to make or break your plans. You can either persevere and realize that obstacles and events are temporary and focus on the future, or you can make it harder on yourself by focusing on the negative. Do yourself a favor and listen to your body, enjoy the positive results and take control of your life.

Book 5: Intermittent Fasting for Women

How to Eat What You Want and Still Lose Weight While on a Budget

By

Beatrice Anahata

Introduction

Congratulations on grabbing your copy of *Intermittent Fasting for Women: How to Eat What You Want and Still Lose Weight While on a Budget* and thank you for doing so.

The following chapters will discuss the different types of safe intermittent fasting methods, and how to shop on even the slimmest of budgets. It is full of tips on how to eat healthy, exercise, and still save money while making the lifestyle change to intermittent fasting.

There are plenty of books on this subject on the market, thanks again for choosing this one! Every effort was made to ensure it is full of as much useful information as possible, please enjoy!

Chapter 1: Fasting Can Be Your New Normal

The word fasting does not exactly conjure happy thoughts, you might even feel your stomach growling just thinking about going a long time without food. However, that is not really the case; there is no reason you have to go long periods without food. Instead, there are many different methods of fasting for you to choose from that will allow you to find the one that works best for both your lifestyle and your body. As you read about the different methods, think about which one jumps out at you, the one that you think would fit into your life the best. Also rule out which ones you think definitely wouldn't. No two people are alike and if something sounds absolutely terrible to you, chances are it would be. So be realistic. There are many options to choose from, and remember, it is a lifestyle change and some discomfort is only natural.

It is important to know that the female body does react different in ways than a male's body. That is because there are different types of hormones that are active in a woman's body to make sure all systems are behaving and performing properly. The biggest and first thing the body will sacrifice when it feels as though it is in starvation mode is the reproductive system. You don't want this to happen, so it is important to follow the rules of the fasting methods and not push yourself too hard. You want to safely reduce your caloric intake, not hurt yourself. That is why you want to do this safely and in a way that works with your body instead of against it. Remember, this is not a one size-fits-all type of deal, you are in complete control of how you choose to fast.

Intermittent fasting simply means not consuming food for a predetermined period of time, generally between twelve to 48 hours. Many people call this time the "fasting period", and what you do consume during this time is completely up to you. For instance, some people decide to only drink water during their fasting period, while others add black coffee, herbal tea, or even different types of bone broth. What you do decide to consume during this time is your choice; even if someone you know only drinks water, do not feel like you need to do the same. Everyone is different, and you might be happier if you get to enjoy your morning cup of coffee, or if you would like to drink green tea throughout the day. At the end of the day, this is your fast, your body, and the goal of fasting is not to make you feel miserable.

Some people think that you are not able to exercise while intermittent fasting, but this is simply not true. There are going to be days and times when you are able to eat normally, and this also means you can and should exercise normally as well. Should you choose the method that requires you to fast for a full 24-hour period, or drastically reduce your caloric intake, don't choose those days to exercise too hard. Instead, do lighter exercises on these days and don't force yourself to work too hard to the point of exhaustion or pain.

How Fasting Works

After you eat, the body spends hours processing the food and burns what it can of the meal you ate. This means that your body has all of it; easily available fuel to burn to create energy. This means that your body will use the food that you just ate to burn instead of stored fat. As you probably know, in order to lose weight, you need to burn fat stores, not just the food you just consumed. This holds especially true if you ate a lot of carbohydrates and sugars because the body will burn sugar before anything else. Keep that in mind when you are eating, because even though you have gone hours during your fasting time, you do not want to overdo it when you do eat by eating too many carbohydrates and sugars.

Of course, this does not mean that you need to give up everything you love. As a matter of fact, nearly everything is fine in moderation. When you are fasting, your body has not only burned off your last meal, but it has also moved passed that and started to burn off fat stores, which is the key to losing weight. Some people think that, because they fast, they are going to want to eat twice as much when they do eat, but that is not the case. Granted, sometimes your meals are going to be a little larger than the meals you had before you began fasting, but your body will adjust rather quickly, and you will find that you are full even though you have skipped a meal or two.

Fasting Methods

Crescendo Method: This is a great introduction to fasting because it does not affect your hormones and does not have a negative impact on your body. Basically, it does not shock the body's systems. The secret to this method of fasting is the schedule and shorter fasting hours. The Crescendo method can also be tailored to fit into your lifestyle, for instance, you fast two or three non-consecutive days each week. On these days, you will fast for between twelve and sixteen hours, again you get to choose the amount of hours that work for you. For instance, sixteen hours might seem too long and, but fourteen fits better into your lifestyle and does not make you miserable.

These hours do not need to be during peak hours of activity either. Most people choose to stop eating at 7:00 p.m. and fast until 9:00 a.m. the next morning. This is just one example. Beginning your fast at 5:00 p.m. and ending it at 7:00 a.m. might work better for you and so on. Just make sure you choose non-consecutive days and that you begin and end your fast at the same times on each of these days every week. Continuity is important because you want your body to adjust, and constantly changing the times is not going to help your body, it will only set you back.

The Crescendo method is also effective because you will be fasting for shorter, less frequent periods of time, while still decreasing your general caloric intake, but preventing the body from going into starvation mode. Keep in mind that this is still a different way of eating, and in the beginning your body is probably going to go through a rebellious phase. This does not mean it is in starvation mode, it is just something new that it needs to adjust to, and it will given time and patience.

16/8 Method: This is one of the most common methods of fasting. It is not a dip your into fasting method though, it is a bit more intense than the Crescendo method, but it does yield results. The 16/8 method means that the 24-hour day is broken up into eight hours and sixteen hours. The eight hours are the eating window and the 16 hours are the fasting period. This is not done only certain days of the week, but every day, which is what makes it a bit more intense. However, it is easy to schedule since you don't have to think about the days of the week, you know which times you are allowed to eat each and every day.

Again, this is not a one-time-fits all method. You get to choose which eight hours to eat and when to fast. One of the most common times is eating from noon to 8:00 p.m., but this might not work for everyone. You can change the times around to suit your lifestyle. You might want to make breakfast a priority, so starting your eating period at 8:00 a.m. and beginning your fasting period at 4:00 p.m., this might seem difficult, but it is up to you. This method can also work for people who work night shifts, which is one the reasons it is so popular since there is so much freedom to choose the fasting and eating times. So, for those people who work throughout the night, their eating times can begin at midnight and end at 8:00 a.m. so it fits into their lifestyle, since they will do their sleeping during the daytime hours. Other diets do not take into the consideration the large amount of people who live a less traditional time-based lifestyle because their sleeping happens mostly during the daylight hours.

Now, once again, even though it is called the 16/8 method, it does not have to be that way. You can even change the times if you choose to, shortening or lengthening by a couple of hours if you need to. Some people choose to do 18/6, meaning they fast for eighteen hours and eat for six, or even 20/4. Do what works for you, just make sure you are continuous in your efforts and give your body time to adjust. The body will not go into starvation mode in sixteen hours, especially since traditionally, nearly half or more of those hours are spent sleeping. Your body is capable of so much, and this is a great way to drastically decrease your caloric intake and burn body fat. Fasting is meant to be a way for the body to burn fat stores, and with this method it most certainly will.

Eat-Stop-Eat Method: This is also a rather common method of fasting because it is used by so many people. It is safe for both men and women and has gained popularity since it can be tailored to fit into so many schedules and lifestyles. This is the one method that does not necessarily require you to stick to such a strict schedule since you can choose the amount of days you want to fast. They do have to be non-consecutive days, but they do not need to be same days each week. With the eat-stop-eat method you simply do not eat for a 24-hour period, two to three days per week.

This is definitely a more intense form of intermittent fasting simply because the body is going to go 24 hours without food, and for some it can incredibly difficult to adjust to. However, the body will still not enter starvation mode from a 24-hour fast. That does not mean that this method is necessarily the easiest either, since the body is accustomed to eating each day. That is why with this fasting method, it is encouraged to drink water and other beverages throughout the day. Many people who practice this method do not restrict their beverage intake on fasting days, enjoying cups of tea, black coffee, and even the very occasional diet soda.

Even though some people do choose to fast three times a week, two is the recommended amount.

The other thing that sets this type of fasting method apart from the others is that people generally refer to their eating days as 'feasting days', not because they get to eat whatever they want in moderation. It is not a good idea for anyone to go overboard with sugars and carbohydrates, and this includes those practicing intermittent fasting, but you can still indulge within reason. The recommended amount of calories for a woman to intake on feasting days is around 2,000 which is more than most traditional diets will allow. Fasting for two 24-hour periods during the week will reduce your caloric intake by around twenty percent, while still allowing you to eat the foods you love.

5:2 Method: This is also called, the 'fast diet'. It is another common form of intermittent fasting for women, but it might not fit into everyone's schedule and it does require counting calories, and for some people that is just not what they are looking for in a fast. Unlike with the other methods, the numbers in the name of the method do not refer to hours, but instead the days of the week. Five days of the week are regular eating days, again, remember that your diet still needs to be rather healthy in order to see results. The other two days of the week, again not two consecutive days, you will consume only 500 to 600 calories.

This means that you will have to pay close attention to the number of calories you are eating on the restricting days. Basically, you want to restrict your caloric intake to a quarter of your traditional intake two days of the week. That is why so many people do prefer this method because there are no full days without eating. A good example of this is to restrict on Mondays and Thursdays, while eating normally throughout the rest of the week. Make sure to eat three small meals on the restricting days and keep close track that each meal not exceed the daily limit when added together. On average, on restricting days meals should be around 200 calories each.

As with the other methods, you can switch the days of the week you want to restrict, just make sure they are the same each week. You can also change the amount of days too, if you choose to. For instance, instead of 5:2, maybe you want to do 4:3, eating normally for four days and restricting for three. Do not exceed more than this though, because this crosses over into dangerous territory and you might end up doing more harm than good, with the most common result being moodiness and weight gain.

Once You Have Made Your Decision

So, you have chosen your method of intermittent fasting, now it's time to actually begin your fast. This is when things can get rather difficult because your body is adjusting to this new way of eating. The first two weeks of any intermittent fasting are difficult, keep that in mind. You might feel like giving up, you might feel like eating anything in site, but this feeling will pass, it just takes time. Remember, there was a time when your body couldn't even consume solid foods, but it learned how. This is the same thing. You need to give your body time to relearn and adjust.

In the beginning you might experience some unfortunate, but common side-effects such as dizziness, irritability, headaches, and even insomnia. Remember, these will pass as they are all part of the process. Your body is learning to burn fat stores and not to simply depend on the meals you have recently consumed since you are going to be either drastically restricting calories or going longer periods of time without consuming calories.

If after two weeks these symptoms persist or get worse, take a step back and reevaluate your chosen method. You might need to choose a different method. Not everyone's body is the same and some fasting methods work better for some and not for others. It might be a simple solution such as switching the fasting days to the days where you are typically less active, or moving around the eating hours to fit into your daily schedule a bit better. So, before giving up, try moving the times around and see how your body reacts to that.

Also, don't forget that you can drink some bone broth or tea to help. This is especially important if you choose to fast for 24-hour periods as this is a difficult method to adjust to. Many people find that drinking tea or coffee also helps them because it makes them feel as though they are not depriving their body of everything. Remember, sometimes the ritual of making coffee or tea is just as important as the consumption of it and depriving your body and brain of that ritual it has come to rely on so heavily can have detrimental effects. So, allow yourself that daily indulgence, just skip the cream and sugar on the fasting days. Some people have a tendency to compare themselves to others, try your best not to do this. Yes, some people can do the eat-stop-eat method and happily consume only water for a 24-hour period, but if you are not one of those people, that's fine. Don't force yourself to be miserable. This is more than just a diet, it is a lifestyle change, and it is not intended to make your life more stressful or to cause you long lasting discomfort.

It is normal for a lifestyle change to be difficult, so listening to your body is important. That's why there are so many different, but still effective methods to choose from. Each person is different, and the way in which someone responds to a certain fast is also going to be different. The people who are most successful at intermittent fasting are the ones who understand that it might take some trial and error. There is no shame in making changes if your first, second, or even third attempt did not work for you.

If you commit to the lifestyle change and make the changes that make it easier for you, you will increase the chances of success. Just like with anything else in life, there is no such thing as instant change or gratification. It is going to take some time for you to see changes, but it will happen. When you are practicing intermittent fasting, you are cutting calories which means you will lose weight. Some of the other added benefits to intermittent fasting include an increase in energy, mental clarity, and even saving money.

When you are first starting your chosen method, it is best to sit down and work out a schedule. You can do this on your phone, a calendar, or even just a piece of paper. Having something in front of you that breaks down the days so you know when your eating and fasting periods are broken down week by week for the entire month, will help put things into perspective. Doing this will also help you schedule personal events and obligations as necessary, because temptation is going to happen, this is especially difficult in the beginning. Sometimes the best thing to do is avoid this until you are more comfortable in your fasting method and your body has adjusted. Doing this will also help increase your chances of success and make the transition to intermittent fasting easier.

Chapter 2: Eat, Just Know When to Do It

Even though you are fasting, you are still going to eat. However, that does not mean that during eating periods you get to eat whatever you want all the time. Just like in everyday life, everything is technically fine, but in moderation. If you fill your body with nothing but over processed foods and sugar during eating periods, you are probably going to gain weight, but this would be true with or without intermittent fasting. The rules for gaining or losing weight do not change. Intermittent fasting is a lifestyle change that is supposed to make it easier to cut out calories because you are eating only during specific times.

For those people who already eat a pretty healthy diet, one that is not full of empty carbohydrates and sugars, this is not going to be too much of a shock to them. However, if you are a fast food, carbohydrate, and sugar lover and that is mostly what your diet consists of, then you are going to need to make more of a lifestyle change than others. You can still eat these things, just learn to limit your intake. Remember, during your eating periods, you still only want to consume around 2,000 calories. It is very easy to go over that limit if you are not paying some attention to what you are eating. The method that requires the most attention to caloric intake is the 5:2 method because for two days you are not to exceed 600 calories at most. This is a low amount of calories and without careful calorie counting, it can be very easy to overdo it and surpass that limit. For some people, they don't want to have to count calories that closely, and that is perfectly okay, that just means that this method is not for them.

Let's assume you chose to go on the 16/8 method, and you have your daily schedule set up. That means each day you have eight hours to eat your 2,000 calories. How you choose to consume those calories is completely up to you. Some people prefer to have the three traditional meals with no snacks in between. Others would rather have two larger meals with some light snacking in between their meals. Just remember that you are not trying to make up for lost calories by eating more calories since you went so long without eating. Don't worry, your body is not going into starvation mode and will actually adjust to this new schedule probably better and easier than you imagined. Again, the first two weeks are going to be the worst and after that, for many people, it simply becomes their regular way of eating and they simply don't think about it anymore.

Dealing with Cravings

For those who have a sweet tooth, you do not have to give up sugar, just make sure to factor it into the allotted amount of calories during your eating periods. Some people will avoid sugar altogether for the majority of their eating periods, and then one day a week indulge in a rich dessert. Others prefer to have a small dessert daily, or during their eating periods, but they make sure to take into consideration that it must be included in their calories.

A common mistake that people make is that they forget that what they are drinking also contains calories. Many people enjoy a good coffee beverage but fail to realize how much sugar is in the drink they order from a coffee shop. The same can be said for sodas, teas, and alcoholic beverages. So, make sure to do some research and find out how many calories are in the things you drink and add them to your caloric intake. Also, some people believe that avoiding all alcohol is best, but some people disagree. This is personal preference, but either way, you must know the calorie consumption and try not to go overboard.

Many people have their own guilty pleasures when it comes to what foods they crave. Intermittent fasting allows you to still indulge, while other diets might cut out foods completely. All you have to do is include the foods you love into the calories that you are consuming and stay within the limit. Of course, this might mean having smaller meals, but sometimes that indulgence means more simply because it can better your mental state. So, if a slice of chocolate cake is something you want, know you might have to make other sacrifices for it in reference to calories, but you can still eat the cake.

Sometimes foods just make us happy because we love them. Of course, there are some people out there who do not really feel this way, but for those people that do, being able to satisfy their craving is incredibly important to them. That is one of the reasons so many people choose intermittent fasting, because it doesn't make them give up the foods they love. It instead teaches them that they can still have it, just some adjustments to the rest of the day's food will need to be made. For so many people, that is a more than fair trade-off and one that they would be happy to make.

Changes Can Be Made

If you are doing the Crescendo method and end your eating period at 5:00 p.m. but find that you are incredibly hungry at 7:00 p.m., simply switch the times so you can allow yourself a small, last snack around 7:00 p.m. You have the power to do that. It might mean that you fast a little longer during the day, but if it works better with your body, then make the necessary changes. The same can be said if you are hungrier early in the morning, simply start your eating period earlier and end it earlier in the day. Some people simply prefer to eat more in the morning and some later in the day. Listen to your body and adjust the times to find what fits best into your lifestyle. Again, this also goes for people with less traditional hours, such as those who work third shift. If you find that you need to eat more late at night before you go to work and less in the morning before you get home and go to sleep, feel free to change your fasting period to accommodate that.

If you want faster, more drastic results, you can also change your eating habits completely, choosing to avoid simple or empty carbohydrates altogether. That's why people who practice the paleo or other keto diets can also benefit from intermittent fasting. If you do choose to do this, try to ease into it. You are already making one big lifestyle change, and to increase your chances of success, change your eating habits slowly. For instance, first just eliminate white bread and pasta from your diet and substitute wheat. Instead of eating a fast food burger, make one at home and use a wheat bun. These are rather small changes that can lead to big results. One of the best forms of motivation is seeing the results of your hard work. Making these changes will lead to the positive changes you want to see which in turn will only want to make you continue.

Some people find that it is also easier to begin their eating period in the middle of the day, so they have time to eat at work and at home. This is especially important for those people who want to save money since this gives them the opportunity to both bring their own lunch and cook their own dinner. Groceries are cheaper than getting takeout and going to a restaurant. Cooking your own food and meal prepping also allows you to easily calculate how many calories you are consuming because you know exactly what is going into each meal.

Fixing Your Times

Some people might find that when doing the 5:2 method, including a weekend day as a fasting period, works best for them because they have that day off work completely. They can use this time to relax and find it easier to not eat when they have less obligations. Other people might find that having a weekend day as a fasting period ruins their weekend, because that is the time when they would rather go out with friends and being able to eat is important to them during that time.

There is absolutely nothing wrong with switching the days around if your first attempt didn't work out for you. Just simply switch the days until you do find a schedule that works for you. Just remember, you cannot fast for two consecutive days, so make sure to give yourself some time in between to refuel and give your body time to process what you have consumed. Your goal is to burn not only what you have recently eaten, but also some of the fat stores on your body, so take that into consideration also when you are making your fasting schedule.

Fasting on days when you are particularly active works for some because they find that it is easier to keep food off their minds when they have so many other things to focus on. Others find that fasting on these days is more difficult because they are just hungrier after doing so much. You don't want your body to feel exhausted and hungry all the time, so if you feel this way, it's time to reevaluate your schedule. Sit down and write out your normal plans for the week and try to schedule your fasting periods on the days when you are not as active. Doing this will make it easier on you and make your body feel better as well. The same goes for the reverse. If you think it would be easier to fast on days when you are more busy and you currently have your fasting period during your more less active times, switch it around. This cannot be stressed enough. Everyone is different and finding what works for you is the most important part of the process.

Sometimes a great place to start is asking yourself which is the most important meal of the day to you, it can be different for everyone. Once you know your answer, you can schedule your eating period to include that meal. If you are doing the 5:2 method, then you can also make that meal the heaviest in calories so you don't feel deprived of your favorite or most important meal. By doing this, you are not only going to feel better physically, but also mentally. Most people don't realize that it is not only the food that makes us happy, but also the ways in which we eat it. The example used earlier was preparing coffee in the morning. For some people, it is what helps them start their day, and going without the caffeine and traditional ritual can have detrimental effects to their mental state. That is what you want to avoid during a fast. If preparing an elaborate dinner is what makes you feel like you have a calm and relaxing end to your day, do not deny yourself of this, simply make it a priority when it comes to your fasting schedule.

This is not going to be an easy journey, especially in the beginning, but you can do it. Patience is key. Give both your mind and body time to adapt to this new schedule you are putting into place. Our bodies know how to burn fuel, and it can adjust to burning fat stores when needed, as long as it does not feel as though it is in starvation mode. Following the methods and sticking to the schedule will prevent this from happening and provide you with the results you want. If you have been sticking to your fasting schedule and are not seeing the results you wanted, you also have the option of eating cleaner or cutting out carbs. There are so many ways to tweak intermittent fasting to make it work for everyone.

Chapter 3: Fasting is On a Schedule, Use it to Save Money

The beauty of intermittent fasting is that you can decide when your fasting periods begin and end so there are no surprises. The same can't be said for other diets that require you to count calories or cut out all carbs. Having a set schedule makes it easy to plan your meals around your fasting periods, and no matter what type of method you are using, you can also meal plan or even take it a step further and meal prep to take all the guessing out of what you are going to eat, saving yourself even more money. In general, though, fasting means you are going to be eating less in general, so either way, you are going to save money.

It's no surprise that cooking at home is cheaper than going to restaurants, if done right, it can also be a lot healthier too. Food and restaurant advertising can feel overwhelming and make you feel that near constant eating is normal. That, of course, is not true. The human body is not built to eat all the time. Our culture is not also based around intermittent fasting either, so this is going to be one of the times in your life when you are going against the grain. Even though this can seem daunting, there is a level of freedom in knowing that you are paving your own way and listening to what your body is telling you, instead of doing what you think you should be doing. Many people are going to assume that you are starving yourself for a certain amount of time and some might caution or give you flack for your 'diet' choice. Remember, this is not a diet, this is a lifestyle and you already fast for a certain number of hours when you sleep. You are simply taking more control of your eating and fasting periods which helps you lose weight, gain mental clarity, and increase focus.

For most people who are trying to lose weight by using intermittent fasting, they treat it as a way for them to eat what they want, just not too much of it. Believe it or not, there is a connection between the way you spend money and the way you consume food. This connection is less based on the financial, and tends to actually have more emotional, almost irrational parallel. For instance, buying or ordering more than what you actually need. Many people find that when checking their bank account history, their food spending mirrored that of their emotional state at the time; it could peak and fall corresponding to someone's mood. This is the opposite of a schedule, and as things tend to be when led by emotion, unpredictable and in the case of food, more expensive than it needs to be.

Some of the common reasons people eat more than they need to can be connected to boredom, negative emotions, stress, or simply because they feel as though they need to. Intermittent fasting helps to end this way of thinking. Intermittent fasting allows you to treat eating as a chance to refuel, to let your body process and digest not only your last meal, but also fat stores. If you find yourself as an emotional or stress eater, then intermittent fasting is really going to benefit you.

Sometimes, we trick ourselves into thinking we need something when we actually don't, and in terms of food, this is not good for the body or the wallet. Think of intermittent fasting as giving yourself a new perspective. You are now going to think in terms of what you actually need and not what you want. Taking away the emotional aspect and replacing it with a strict schedule and foods that you need, is definitely going to cause some discomfort, but it will definitely be worth it. When you begin your chosen method of intermittent fasting, try to think about what you are getting, and not what you are missing. This definitely sounds easier said than done, but you are still going to be able to have moments of indulgence. There are just going to be fewer of them, and your body will thank you for it.

For those who are already on a tight budget and think that intermittent fasting is going to be too expensive, that couldn't be further from the truth. You are consuming fewer calories while intermittent fasting, meaning you are eating less, which in turn means you spend less on what you do eat. People

338

have different reasons for intermittent fasting, and finding out why you are doing it and what you want to get out of it is going to help you succeed. So, start off by making a list of what you want to achieve through intermittent fasting as it will help you decide what you want to eat. Some people do not want to cook at home. For those people, it is still possible to save money because they too are going to go longer periods of time without eating.

If you do decide to most of your eating from restaurants, start asking how many calories are in the meals you eat. This is especially important if you are on the 5:2 method, because you do have strict limits for two days of the week. If you don't stick to the method of your choice, then you will not see any benefits, and not paying attention to the amount of calories that are in the foods you eat, you are going to set yourself back.

A New Schedule

Even though you probably think that you are going to be miserable from not eating, you will quickly find out that it is not the case. Intermittent fasting allows you to simplify your life. Think about how much time you spend, not just eating, but thinking about what to eat. Going longer times without eating means less stress and time spent worrying about what to eat. Many people are surprised by how much time went into food related matters and are amazed how much time is freed up when they begin their intermittent fasting lifestyle.

It is this newly acquired free time that gives you the freedom to accomplish more, it's almost like your days get longer. Suddenly, you have more time during the day to get work done, exercise, or simply relax. When you first begin your fasting method, it is a good idea to occupy your free time by keeping busy. There is definitely an adjust period, and it can be uncomfortable adapting to a new eating period. If you keep yourself busy, it can help keep your mind off of the fact that you might be hungry when your fasting period begins. This is one of the reasons so many people who practice intermittent fasting also take time to create a detailed grocery list to further reduce food related stress, and as yet another way to just simplify their lives.

You are probably going to notice an increase in your focus, discipline, and overall productivity. That is another one of the reasons people choose to change their lifestyle to include intermittent fasting. How people experience this varies from person to person. For instance, some people claim that they have more alertness in during the day when they skip breakfast and do not start their eating period until later in the day. While some people experience this later in the day, when their eating period has ended. Once you know how your body is going to react to this, you can schedule your important or major events or meetings to correspond with the times in which you feel more focused and alert.

Intermittent fasting requires a level of discipline that you might not have anticipated. This is part of the adjustment process and you will find that your overall discipline will also rise. This generally happens naturally, because you are retraining your brain to act and respond in a different way than it had previously. When you start to make more aware, careful decisions about food, it will simply translate to other aspects of your life. It feels nice to be in control, and intermittent fasting will show you that.

It is in your best interest to set yourself up for success. It is human nature to want to eat foods high in sugars and carbohydrates when your eating period beings after a long period of fasting. Again, it takes a lot of discipline to fast, but it takes even more discipline to eat completely clean and intermittent fast. That's why it is better for your mental health to allow for some indulgences from time to time. Part of setting up success means shopping ahead of time and knowing what you are going to put into your body and when. If your cupboards and refrigerator are full of healthy foods, then that is what you will eat when your fasting period ends.

The same can be said for self-sabotage. Since intermittent fasting does require self-discipline, it can be easy to accidentally overdo it with the calories. Of course, this doesn't mean that you need to eat clean all the time, but it does mean that you need put forth the effort to find out how many calories are in what you're eating. Some of the ways to help you prevent this from happening are to spread meals and snacks out during your eating period if your body responds better to that type of diet. If your body responds to two larger meals to feel satiated, then you can do it that way too. It's important to listen to your body and make changes accordingly.

Learning to listen to your body is one of the hardest parts of intermittent fasting since many people are accustomed to eating when they feel like it or when others are eating. So much of our lives revolve around food that many people have stopped listening to their bodies and started listening to what is around them, regardless of if they are actually hungry or not. This is a hard habit to break. One of the easiest places to start is to grocery shop when you are not hungry. This seems like common sense, but even people who are not intermittent fasting make this mistake. When you shop while hungry, you are more likely to throw unhealthy and over processed food into your cart because that is what you're craving at the moment.

Not only will this hurt your body, but it will also be harder on your wallet. Shopping smart doesn't just involve not shopping while hungry, it also means having a general idea of what you are going to buy before you go. This will make it easier to make healthy choices. Some people choose to meal plan or prep and make the same things each week, but this just personal preference and not something that you have to do, it is completely up to you. Finding what works for you can also be fun, try not to be too hard on yourself. You are making a lifestyle change. That means that you still need to live your life. Finding your stride and balance between fasting and living your life will happen, it just takes time and patience.

As you start your fasting journey remember to listen to your body. For some people, it has been a long time since they have done this in terms of food. However, this is the best way to ensure your success. Your body can and will tell you what it needs. That doesn't mean your body won't fight you when it is adapting to this new schedule of eating, but with time and discipline, both your mind and body will adapt, and you will reap the benefits. The unknown is scary for many people, so is intermittent fasting, because it is something they have not done previously. This is common and fortunately, it is short lived since intermittent fasting is not what many people expect, and the body is capable of more than what many people ask of it.

Chapter 4: Caloric Intake and Fasting

Many diets require you to reduce the amount of calories you consume by only allowing you to eat certain food. Granted, you are going to lose weight if you restrict calories, but you might also be miserable by doing so since you can't eat the foods you love. Even if you don't want to admit it, there are some foods that just make you feel better, whether it be chocolate cake or macaroni and cheese. You are only human, and there is nothing wrong with enjoying your food. Some diets make it nearly impossible to enjoy the foods you love, but intermittent fasting is not one of them.

It is simple math: if you reduce the calories you consume and still exercise the same amount or more than before, you will lose weight. Intermittent fasting reduces caloric intake by reducing the amount of time you are able to eat. It isn't that you are eating smaller meals or cutting out sugar or carbohydrates altogether, instead you are skipping meals completely and in doing so reducing your caloric intake. It's simple really, not eating for longer period of time means the hard work is done for you. No food was consumed, therefore your daily and weekly calorie count is lower.

Intermittent fasting is actually one of the least complex eating methods, which is one of the reasons it has gained so much in popularity. The beauty is in its simplicity. There are no points to keep track of, no carbohydrates to cut out, unless of course, you choose to. You probably think that you will want to binge once you begin your eating period after fasting, and at first you might, but this will change with just a little bit of time and discipline. Each method of fasting requires you to consume a healthy 2,000 calories during normal eating periods, and either no calories or very little during other times.

What you decide to eat during your eating period is up to you, but if you want the best results, choosing to fill those 2,000 calories with healthy, whole foods is going give you faster, more drastic results. Either way though, intermittent fasting still reduces stomach fat, and will only do it better and more quickly if you do decide to eat healthier. A flat stomach has more to do with what you eat and less to do with exercise. People are often surprised to hear this, but it is especially true for women. That's why intermittent fasting reduces stomach fat so quickly, because this is the type of food that begins with the food and a caloric deficit will show in stomach weight first for most women.

As long as you stick to your chosen method and do not exceed the 2,000 calories, you will automatically achieve a caloric deficit, which is the key to losing weight. Skipping entire meals reduces the amount of calories you eat, so much that you don't really have to worry too much about the calories you do eat when your fasting period is over. For example, if you eat peanut butter, toast, and a glass of orange juice in the morning, this by itself is around 500 calories. Some people also have a morning or midmorning tea or coffee beverage that can contain up to 150 calories, for instance, the average latte contains around 130. If you were to fast in the morning and not start eating until around lunch time, you are cutting out nearly 700 calories.

If a woman eats between 1,600 to 2,000 calories per day, just skipping that one meal is between twenty to almost thirty percent of their caloric intake saved instantly. Then, later in the day, if you ate two larger meals that are around 750 calories each, and a dessert around 300 calories, you are still only consuming 1,800 calories which is well on the way to weight loss. Even better is that you do not have to give up anything that you love. This is about changing the times that you eat, not what you eat.

Intermittent fasting is also one of the easiest ways to burn actual fat. For instance, when you start a low carbohydrate diet, the number on the scale will drop quickly, but you are losing water from your body, not real fat. Sometimes, you can also cut calories so much that the body will actually hold onto fat cells and burn muscle as an alternative source of fuel. This is what happens when the body goes into starvation mode, and that is what you want to avoid. Intermittent fasting, when done properly, will not cause you to lose muscle mass. Your body will not feel like it is going into starvation and will burn fat stores to use as energy. This is how you lose weight and keep it off.

If you find yourself losing muscle mass or not seeing the desired results, you can and should tweak your fasting times or caloric intake. As mentioned before, the best way to gauge this is to listen to your body. There are different types of intermittent fasting for a reason. Not everyone is built the same and everyone's body responds differently. That's why you can change the times to match what works for you. Just make sure not to go too far above an average healthy caloric intake, or too far below it either, since that can be just as harmful. The key is to be patient and listen to your body, but don't be too strict, this isn't meant to make you miserable and moody, which can happen if you aren't being safe.

What you put into your body when you do eat is completely your choice. As you have seen, skipping meals already gives you an edge with the caloric deficit, but you can take it a step further and choose to eat very healthy when your eating period begins. Of course, this is not going to be easy as the body is going to feel run down and craving foods rich in carbohydrates and sugar. However, you can eat a lot more vegetables and fruits than sugary and carbohydrate heavy foods, meaning you will feel fuller while eating less calories. Some people choose to do this because it frees them up to have more snacks during their eating period or allows them to have a more calorie heavy dessert.

You also have to remember that it is important to burn calories too, and in the beginning the last thing you are going to want to do is exercise, especially during your fasting period. That is perfectly fine. It is actually recommended to do light exercise while fasting, but some people prefer to do heavier workouts during a fasting period. Only do what your body can handle, there is no one right way to fast intermittently. What works for one person might not work for another. The same goes for exercising and fasting, it might take some trial and error before you figure out what works well for you. Some people try to keep up with their regular exercise routines but find that it is too intense during their fasting period. If you feel this way, lighten up your workout on fasting days if you are doing the 5:2 or eat-stop-eat method. If you are doing any of the other methods, you can learn to plan your workouts around your food intake times.

One of the most common things that people do is to plan their eating times around their workouts, or vice versa. After a workout the body is typically very hungry, and hard workouts and fasting can be a recipe for failure. You can prevent this from happening by working out based on your eating period. Exercise when you still have time to eat afterwards if that is how your body operates. On the other hand, if your body works better with a larger meal before a heavy workout, cater to it that way.

Most people plan their food out based on how it makes them feel in terms of their energy levels throughout the day, which includes their exercise routine. They want to feel their best which serves as natural motivation to eat healthier, because it keeps them from feeling sluggish during the day and lets them workout harder. Generally, this comes with time and experience, because everyone is different. Some people might find that they prefer to eat a high carbohydrate vegetarian diet, while others prefer a low carbohydrate, but higher fat and protein diet to feel their best. Eat when and what works for you but be consistent. Your diet and fast doesn't have to match someone else's, but you won't see the results and reap the benefits of intermittent fasting if you are not consistent with what works for you.

If you are doing the eat-stop-eat method, then you are going a full 24 hours without eating, two to three times each week. For fasts that are long like that, it is a good idea to use those days to do light exercise or as resting days. If you do choose to do some form of exercise on these days, begin with some light exercises to see how your body responds before you jump into a heavier workout. A good example of some exercises to do include: yoga, speed walking, swimming, and anything else that is relatively low impact. If you do not feel light headed or dizzy from this, continue to increase your workouts until you see fit, as long as you stop if you feel any detrimental side-effects of the workouts.

You do not have to stick to the 2,000 calories a day either, you can safely drop to 1,600 as that is a healthy amount too. The 2,000 calorie is an average, and for those who are trying to lose weight, it would be more beneficial for them to stick to a 1,600 calorie a day diet. You can always adjust your caloric intake as you go depending on the results you are seeing. It's helpful to also know that once you reach a healthy weight, your body will naturally maintain it and weight loss will slow down. This usually happens after a year or so of intermittent fasting, and one of the reasons it is so effective is because it takes very little to maintain a healthy weight. It is also another reason that intermittent fasting is considered a lifestyle and not a diet, because once you have made it a habit, it feels natural and becomes your new normal.

Just remember that intermittent fasting is not meant to feel like torture, of course it is going to take some time to adjust to, but if after a few weeks you feel tired and rundown, make some changes. You have the power to change nearly everything about how you fast, as long as you follow the basic rules and always take your safety into consideration. You do not have to give up the chocolate you love so much, or not train for the marathon you've been looking forward to. In fact, you can still eat what you want, exercise normally, and still manage to either lose weight or maintain a healthy weight.

The hardest part of this journey is going to be the beginning. Many people find they don't really know where to start, or how to begin. There is no secret, you just have to do it. That's it. Sure, you might stumble or break your fast before you're supposed to sometimes, but just try again the next day and make changes if you feel you need to. Your body knows what it's doing, it's your job to listen to it, and intermittent fasting is a great way to learn to do that. So, don't be afraid to make some mistakes, it's the best way to learn sometimes. You need to know what not to do to find what works for you sometimes, and that's okay.

Chapter 5: Save Money, Make a Grocery List

You already know that you are going to be eating less, an entire meal is going to be left out of your diet. That means that you get to spend less at the grocery store too. For instance, if you begin your eating period around lunch and continue through dinner, that means that you are not eating breakfast. Consider, it a thing of the past. Not only is it something that you don't have to worry about anymore, but it's also something that you don't have to pay for anymore either. This frees you up to just buy lunch, dinner, snack, and dessert foods, most of which are interchangeable. Of course, the exception to this is the 5:2 and the eat-stop-eat methods where you are eating all three meals on other days, but significantly cutting calories on the other two days, or fasting altogether.

Regardless of the method that you chose, the best thing you can do to save money is to cook at home and meal prep. Not only does this reduce the stress of wondering what you are going to eat, it also means that you can make a plan which will help you make better choices. Of course, you do not have to do it this way, but it can really help to simplify your life and get the most benefits from intermittent fasting. You are probably thinking about how much more expensive it is to eat healthier foods, when processed, prepackaged, or takeout is so much cheaper. Well, sometimes that may be true, there are some things that you can do to eat healthier even on the super tight budget.

Tips to Shopping on a Budget – And Keep It Healthy

- Work with your environment and the season. Fruits and vegetables that are in season are cheaper than their counterparts that are transported from farther away. So, feel free to stock up on the cheaper fruits and veggies and then freeze them to use later. Make sure to label everything with the date and check to see how long it will keep when frozen, since some items keep longer than others. You can also prep smoothies in this way too, so all you have to do is throw them in the blender with some yogurt or milk if you prefer for a healthy snack or dessert.

- Shop smart. If your grocery store or co-op has a member card that gives discounts, get it. Also, check the circulars and shop what is on sale. This will be a great way to create variety since sales change so often. One of the best ways to save money is to be buy the protein that is on sale that week and plan your meals around that. You might be eating a lot of fish or chicken in one week, but it will be cheaper than going out or not buying what it is on sale. Plus, it can be a fun way to learn to cook things you didn't know how to before. The internet is a wonderful place to find healthy recipes. It doesn't matter if you are vegan or meat eater, you can find something interesting to make with the ingredients that are on sale.

- Speaking of meat, get a little adventurous with the cuts that you get. Obviously, some are more expensive than others, so go with a cheaper cut. You are intermittent fasting after all, consuming less calories is par for the course. You can add a little bit of a fattier cut of meat into your diet. Also, bone-in, tougher cuts, and skin-on cuts are all going to be cheaper. If you are feeling even more adventurous, organs are also incredibly cheap and are nutritious and flavorful. This is also another great opportunity to explore less traditional recipes online. Another great rule of thumb when it comes to tougher cuts of meat in general, don't forget to bring out the crockpot.

Sometimes, that is the secret to making even the toughest cuts delicious and healthy.

- If you are vegan or vegetarian, you are no stranger to different types of beans and grains. However, if it's new to you, learn to embrace whole grains and substitute beans for meat in your meals throughout the week. Beans are cheaper than meat and are also nutritious. Avoid white bread if you can, since it is empty carbohydrates and provides very little nutritional value and opt for the whole wheat bread that is on sale instead. Sometimes, there is a manager's special in the bakery department on breads that are a little older. So, don't forget to check there, and don't be shy to ask someone who works there if you can't find it easily. Other cheap grains are freekeh, brown rice, and quinoa.

- Explore foods from other cultures, for instance, Mexican food relies heavily on rice and beans. Use brown rice as a healthy and cheap alternative. Indian food is another flavorful and healthy option. If you think that you don't like Indian or Mexican food, look up different recipes online, chances are you just haven't found the right dish yet. Or it might not be the entire entrée that you don't like, but a specific herb or spice. An example is that, to some people, cilantro tastes like soap. So just keep trying until you find something you like. Don't be scared to tweak recipes that you find to make them more personally palatable.

- This should probably go without saying, but keep your kitchen organized. Know what ingredients you are out of, or running low on. It can be difficult to eat healthy after a day of long, hard work, only to come home and find out that you are out of chicken, or quinoa. That's when the temptation to order unhealthy takeout might win. This is another reason meal planning is so important; it will prevent issues like this from occurring. If you keep an organized kitchen and have a specific plan set out that includes everything you need to eat for the week, down to each ingredient, then the more likely you are to have everything and eat healthier.

- One of the greatest ways to save money is to reduce waste. You can do this by getting creative and repurposing your leftovers. Again, the internet is a wonderful place to find recipes for nearly anything. For instance, if you bake a chicken, you cannot only use the bones to create your own bone broth, but you can also use any of the leftover meat to make a soup or even a healthy wrap for lunch the next day. Don't throw food away if you think you can make something with it later. You can even freeze items if you think you can use them later.

- Shop at other places. There is no reason that you have to do all of your shopping at the same store unless you want to. Different stores are going to have different sales for you to take advantage of, and swing by your local farmer's market right before they close. Vendors are more likely to give you a good deal just so they don't have to transport it back and forth.

- Another option is bargaining, and bargain bins for ugly produce. These are the fruits and vegetables that are slightly bruised or nearly overripe. They are often highly discounted at stores. You can also ask the local farmer's market vendor to sell you their 'ugly' produce for cheaper. More often than not it gets thrown away, making your chances of getting it for cheap even higher.

- Check out your local ethnic markets too, you will be surprised what you find there at bargain prices. Also, you can find some interesting proteins, fruits, and vegetables too, usually at very reasonable prices. For instance, rice noodles in a traditional grocery store can be expensive, but at an Asian market they are much cheaper.

- Don't be afraid to try new things. Remember to keep an open mind when you are wondering around different places. Just because you haven't had something before, doesn't mean it's bad. It probably just means you are going to have to learn to prepare it properly and figure out how to work into your meal planning. Some of the best things come from happy accidents. Stumbling upon interesting and unique ingredients are no exception.

- The most important tip of all, again, try not to go grocery shopping while you're hungry. Your hunger is going to prevent you from making sound, healthy decisions, and if you have the power to prevent that, do it. If you have no other option, make a detailed list and try your best to stick it.

Meal prepping is going to be the easiest choice, since you can make a detailed grocery list mapping out everything you are going to eat or drink during the week. However, this method is not for everyone. For those people who hate to cook or who just prefer takeout and restaurants, there's nothing wrong with that as long as you also make healthy choices. The key to this is going to be communication. Act like you are shopping for your food and don't be shy about asking what ingredients are in the food you are ordering, as well as the calorie count. A good rule of thumb: if there is no way to determine how many calories are in an entrée, don't order it. You can always look things up online, but to do so accurately, you need to know the amount of the different ingredients.

It doesn't matter if you are shopping for yourself or ordering out, your goal is to make good decisions. When you prefer to not cook at home, it can take some creativity as well. For instance, get familiar with the ala carte menu at your favorite restaurants. The portions are generally listed, and you can look up your caloric intake online if you need to. Also, branch out, try different types of restaurants such as Turkish, Ethiopian, or even Vietnamese if you haven't had it before. There are a lot of new and fun healthy options out there. These types of restaurants can also be much cheaper too.

If you find that you are spending too much money from eating out, then you can do a combination of cooking at home and going out. Many people will meal plan and prep for the weekdays and allow their weekends to be a bit more spontaneous so they can go out with friends. If this is the method you choose, don't forget to check the calories. You need to have some idea, just so you know how much you can eat or drink later.

This brings us to adult beverages. Some people are going to say to abstain from them altogether, while others are going to say it's fine in moderation. Just be sure to add the calories from your drinks into your daily intake and avoid them altogether during fasting periods. This is completely personal preference. If you want to forgo dessert in favor of a glass of wine or a cocktail, do it. Again, not only is this your life, but your fast, and you are free to do as you please. Of course, remember that alcohol does have sugar in it and it is not going to help in weight loss. But knowing what you know, if you still want that glass of wine, make the necessary sacrifice other calories from something else and enjoy.

No matter which method you choose, or what you decide to eat, you are making a decision for yourself and taking your eating schedule into your own hands. It might not always be easy, but few things worth it ever are. Your hard work, dedication, and discipline will pay off in the end! So, just keep going, be patient with yourself, and learn from your mistakes. You're allowed to make mistakes and learn from them, it's part of the process when there is no one-size-fits-all fasting method. So, don't be too hard on yourself and remember to have some fun.

Book 6: Intermittent Fasting

*The 30-Day Fat Shredding Meal Plan
to Building More Muscle, Staying Lean
and Getting Healthy.*

By

Beatrice Anahata

Introduction

If you have already heard of intermittent fasting, you are likely aware of many of the benefits that this method of eating can provide. If you are new to the concept of intermittent fasting, here are the basics!

Intermittent fasting is a natural way of eating that more accurately follows the way humans ate hundreds or thousands of years ago. The constant availability of food that we experience in today's society is a new phenomenon. Think back to only a century ago: many people grew their own crops, raised their own animals, and spent a lot of time preserving food for the winter season. They could not simply stop by the grocery store when they ran out of food. Once a certain food was gone, they had to wait until they could grow, raise, or preserve it again. Constant snacking was not possible because food had to be eaten mindfully. It was important to keep enough food to survive until spring. Looking even farther back in time to when humans were hunter-gatherers, we find a similar pattern. People had to work hard to find their food, by hunting fish and game or collecting berries and plants. Sometimes they had to go long periods without food because they could not find anything to eat. As a result of this history, the human body is well-adapted to a style of eating that includes periods of fasting, and poorly adapted to the constant availability of food that we experience today. Intermittent fasting reawakens the body's natural capabilities to store and use its own energy reserves, resulting in weight loss, increased energy, and a better lifestyle. It's the polar opposite of many popular diet programs! In addition, intermittent fasting doesn't require that you eat specially prepared meals or specific diet foods. In some cases (such as the Warrior Diet), following a meal plan can be very beneficial in addition to intermittent fasting. However, in most cases, you can eat the same foods as you have always eaten. It is only the timing and frequency of the meals that will change.

The most important consideration when it comes to intermittent fasting is choosing which plan is right for you. You should keep several considerations in mind when choosing a plan. First and most importantly, does the plan fit into your lifestyle? Many diets involve radical changes in lifestyle that make them difficult to follow. Losing weight is hard enough without having to make huge changes in your everyday life. This is especially true when many diet plans seem to have been designed for people with endless energy and lots of free time. Some people do have time and energy to spare, but many of us have busy lives. When we come home at the end of the day, cooking and working out are not high on our list of priorities! Intermittent fasting solves many of these problems because it doesn't require radical changes.

Nevertheless, each method of intermittent fasting is a little different. When choosing a method to try, think about your daily habits. What are your work hours? When are you most busy? When do you like to relax? Do you have days off on weekends? What about during the week? What do you like to do with your free time? These considerations will help you pick the intermittent fasting method that is the best fit for you. You can always try several different methods if you are unsure, then make your decision based on experience.

This will be a modified Intermittent Fasting schedule with a few other days mixed in such as flush days and Low carb days. This will allow you to mix in a different eating schedules every 3 days out of the week. On the days you do intermittent fasting you will consume 40% of your calories from a healthy protein source (chicken, fish, steak, turkey burger), 35% will come from healthy fat sources (avocado, olives, and olive oil, walnuts, soybeans, coconut oil, flaxseed, sunflower seeds) and 25% from Carbohydrates (sweet potato, quinoa).

You will be eating more fruits and vegetables than what you are typically used to. These are loaded with vitamins, minerals, phytochemicals, and fiber. Consuming these foods will allow you to feel fuller for longer as well. Regulation of insulin will be closely linked to the consumption of fruits and vegetables and insulin extracts the nutrients needed from the blood stream and diverts it to the surrounding tissues.

What is intermittent fasting?

A type of scheduled eating plan where you simply restrict your normal daily eating to a 6-8 hour window of time without cutting calories. You will still consume 2-3 meals within this window to fulfill your calorie allotment.

Morning time is the best time to burn fat. When you wake up you are in a fasted state. Your body is currently in a low insulin state and is an ideal time for the body to dip into its fat stores.

Intermittent fasting has been shown to lower insulin and increase FFAs more than any other diet or calorie restriction plan.

What are the benefits of intermittent fasting?

1. Increases insulin sensitivity

2. Reduces inflammation

3. Increases blood sugar control

4. Decreases blood pressure

5. Increases fatty acid oxidation (fat burning)

6. Decreases cholesterol and stress

7. Increases cellular repair

8. Peaked performance in sports and activities

How does it work?

- From 0-6 hours your body is using energy from its last meal.
- From 6-14 hours your body is using its blood glucose.
- From 14-16 hours your body is in fat burning mode.
- From 16-24 hours your body is in full blown fat burning mode and this is the best time to workout.

Cans & Cants

- There will be no sugars or processed foods.
- Your grains and dairy will be limited.
- You CAN consume butter and fruit juice as a sweetener.
- Coffee will be acceptable in moderation.
- Foods with MSG, Sulfites will be avoided.
- Animal proteins+ lots of vegies+ high quality fats+ seasonings=SUCCESS

How will it make me feel?

An empty stomach triggers a cascade of hormonal responses throughout the body conducive to building muscle and burning fat." You're going to be hungry, your stomach will want food and will let you know about it at the same time. This will be a good feeling for you as your body is literally burning off the fat, so as you experience. By the time your first meal rolls around you'll feel like eating a whole horse.

How will this help me?

Exercising while fasting is crucial to your fitness plans as it allows your body to effectively shed fat, thanks to your sympathetic nervous system (SNS), which controls your natural fat-burning processes. SNS is activated by exercise and lack of food. This combination of fasting and exercise maximizes the impact of cellular factors and catalysts (cyclic AMP and AMP Kinases), which force the breakdown of fat and glycogen for energy.

This will be tough, but remember your mind, your goals and your strong determination will get you to your long term goal. Let's go!!

Nutrition Plan

There will be 3 different scheduled eating days including a flush day, moderate carb day and an intermittent fasting day. You will perform a 3-day cycle alternating between all 3 different nutritional days. Females will consume the lower end of the oz. scale (i.e 3-5oz. of chicken) and males with consume the higher end of this scale.

Meal Preparation

Meal Preparation will be a key in your success, look ahead at your week and decide what you will need to prepare for. Examples of this would be to put mixed nuts into baggies, slice any fruits and vegetables, make a list of all food items you will need and do one grocery shopping trip.

Intermittent Fasting Day- You will not be cutting calories as women will consume 1100 and 1500 calories and males 1600-2000 calories. You are required to eat either 14-16 hours after your last meal or typically around 2p.m. You will feed your body all the same calories in a typical eating day within an 8-10-hour window.

Intermittent fasting Day Menu

A typical intermittent fasting day will include eating between 2-5p.m for meal #1 and 5-9p.m for meal #2

Day 1-

Meal #1 2-3 eggs with ½ avocado and 8-10 olives; handful of almonds or walnuts; ½ sweet potato with 4-6oz of chicken and unlimited strips of green peppers.

Meal # 2 1- 1 ½ cups quinoa with ½ avocado and 3-5 oz. fish

Day 2-

Meal #1 Steak and Eggs- (3-5oz steak and 2 - 3eggs with green pepper and spinach; carrots and pepper strips with hummus)

Meal #2 4-6oz Chicken w/ salad and ½ avocado; ½ cup mixed nuts

Day 3-

Meal #1 Layer two rye crisp breads with 1/4 avocado and sliced hard-boiled eggs make 5-6 of these; 1 cup low fat cottage cheese

Meal # 2 Apple and Chicken Curry- (Mix 1 Boneless chicken breast; ¼ cup coconut oil &chicken broth; 1 cubed apple and 1tsb of garlic/curry powder/ginger/olive oil) Cook ½-1 cup brown rice separately and mix together.

**Food substitutions for any day: whole wheat pretzels, baby shrimp, turkey bacon, black beans.

Grocery List

Fruits and Veggies

- Blackberries
- Grapefruit
- Oranges (1 bag)
- Strawberries
- Bananas
- Corn (fresh, canned, or frozen)
- Zucchini (3 small-medium)
- Onion
- Jarred roasted red peppers
- Baby carrots
- Cherry tomatoes (3 cartons)
- Dried fruit (apricots, raisins, craisins, dates, blueberries, bananas, etc.)
- Tomatoes (5-6)
- Apples (1 bag)

- Lettuce (3 bags)
- Spinach (2 bags)
- Pears (2)
- Alfalfa sprouts
- Cucumber (2 medium)
- Limes (2)
- Diced pineapple (1 large can or 2 small cans)
- Frozen peas (1 bag)
- Garlic (1 head)
- Red bell pepper (2)
- Portobello mushrooms (2)
- Eggplant (1 small)
- Avocado (2)
- Artichoke hearts (1 small can)

Dairy/Eggs

- Greek yogurt
- 2% milk
- Eggs
- Butter
- Smoked Gouda
- Individual Greek yogurts (2)
- Fresh mozzarella
- Light cream cheese

- Shredded cheese (mozzarella or any kind)
- Feta cheese (1 small container)

Grains

- Granola (1 box)
- Steel-cut oats
- Whole wheat bread (2 loaves)
- Wheat bran
- Couscous
- Orzo
- Rice (small bag)
- Flour tortillas (small package)
- Gnocchi (1 package)

Baking

- Salt
- Baking powder
- Baking soda
- Brown sugar
- Vanilla
- Wheat flour
- Olive oil

Protein

- Canned tuna (2)
- Salmon fillets (3)
- Halibut (½ lb)
- Tilapia fillets (2)
- Sardines in tomato sauce (1 can)
- Smoked deli ham
- Boneless, skinless chicken breasts (2)
- Chicken thighs (2)
- Chicken breast tenders (5-7)
- Ground beef (¼ lb)

Spices

- Pepper
- Cinnamon
- Cumin (ground)
- Fresh dill
- Fresh mint
- Fresh basil
- Fresh coriander
- Fresh parsley
- Fresh sage
- Ground turmeric
- Garlic powder

- Ground red pepper
- Oregano (fresh or dried)
- Chili powder
- Cilantro (optional)
- Nutmeg (0ptional)

Nuts

- Almonds, salted or unsalted
- Toasted slivered almonds
- Walnuts

Other

- Honey
- Maple syrup
- Mustard
- Cranberry chutney
- Fish sauce
- Lemon juice
- White wine vinegar
- Red wine vinegar
- Balsamic vinegar
- Dry white wine or white cooking wine

- Sweet chili sauce
- Fig preserves
- Potato chips
- Pesto
- Capers
- Salsa verde
- Skewers
- Chicken stock (optional)

30-Day Fat Shredding Meal Plan

Day 1: Non-fast day

Breakfast: Citrus-Blackberry Oatmeal

Ingredients:

Steel-cut oats

2% milk

Blackberries

Grapefruit

Oranges

Directions:

- The evening before, combine ¼ cup uncooked steel-cut oats with ½ cup 2% milk. Place in an airtight container and refrigerate overnight, at least eight hours. In the morning, microwave the oats for thirty seconds. Top with one cup of fresh blackberries and one cup of sliced orange and grapefruit segments.
- Drink water, tea, or coffee.

Lunch: Fancy Tuna Sandwich

Ingredients:

Canned tuna

Olive oil

Jarred roasted red peppers

Fresh basil

Red wine vinegar

Whole wheat bread

Almonds

Directions:

- Drain one can of tuna. Chop ¼ cup roasted red peppers and two tablespoons fresh basil. Mix the tuna, red peppers, and basil with ½ tablespoon olive oil and ½ teaspoon red wine vinegar. Make sandwiches using whole wheat bread.
- As a side, have five baby carrots and five cherry tomatoes. Drink water, tea, or coffee.

Snack: Twenty almonds, salted or unsalted

Dinner: Tomato-Balsamic Salmon with Couscous

Ingredients:

One salmon fillet

Olive oil

Salt

Pepper

Cherry tomatoes

Fresh basil

Onion

Balsamic vinegar

Couscous

Water

Directions:

- Use tinfoil to line a baking sheet. Preheat the oven to 500 degrees Fahrenheit. To make the salmon, combine ⅛ teaspoon salt and ⅛ teaspoon pepper. Sprinkle on the fillet. Heat ½ tablespoon olive oil in a pan. Sear the fillet on one side for four minutes or until golden brown. Place the fillet on the baking sheet, seared side up. Bake another four minutes.

- To make the sauce, pour another ½ tablespoon of olive oil into the pan. Sauté two tablespoons thinly sliced onion for two minutes. Add a sprinkle of salt and pepper, ⅔ cup cherry tomatoes, and two tablespoons roughly chopped fresh basil. Cook another two minutes. Add ½ tablespoon balsamic vinegar and cook for one minute more.

- To make the couscous, heat ½ cup water and a dash of olive oil in a small pot with a tight-fitting lid. When the water boils, pour in ¼ cup couscous, cover, and remove from the heat. Let the pot sit for five minutes until the couscous has absorbed all the water. Fluff with a fork.

- Serve the salmon with a side of couscous, and garnish with the sauce. Have a salad with your favorite dressing as a side. Drink water, tea, or coffee.

Day 2: Non-fast day

Breakfast: Strawberry Parfait

Ingredients:

Greek yogurt

Strawberries

Granola

Toasted slivered almonds

Directions:

- Spoon ¼ cup Greek yogurt into a parfait or sundae glass. Add ¼ cup sliced strawberries and ¼ cup granola. Repeat with another layer of Greek yogurt, strawberries, and granola. Top with two tablespoons toasted slivered almonds.
- Drink water, tea, or coffee.

Lunch: Smoked Ham and Cheese Sammie

Ingredients:

Whole wheat bread

Mustard

Smoked deli ham

Smoked Gouda

Butter

Directions:

- Spread two slices of bread with butter on one side and mustard on the other. Layer smoked deli ham and slices of Gouda on the mustard side of the bread. Cook the sandwich in a hot pan, covered, until the bottom slice of bread is toasted and the cheese is melting. Uncover, flip the sandwich, and cook until the other side is toasted.

- Have a handful of potato chips as a side. Drink water, tea, or coffee.

Snack: Two apples

Dinner: Summery Chicken Tacos

Ingredients:

3 large or 5 small chicken breast tenders

Olive oil

Cumin (ground)

Salt

Pepper

Onion

Corn (fresh, canned, or frozen)

Zucchini

Salsa verde

Cilantro (optional)

Flour tortillas

Shredded cheese (any kind)

Directions:

- Cut the chicken breast tenders into one-inch pieces. Combine ½ teaspoon ground cumin, ⅛ teaspoon salt, and ⅛ teaspoon pepper, then sprinkle over the chicken pieces. Heat ½ tablespoon olive oil in a pan. Add the chicken and cook for three minutes. Next, add ⅓ cup chopped onion, ⅓ cup corn, and ⅓ cup chopped zucchini. Cook for another two minutes, until the chicken is done. Stir in three tablespoons salsa verde and one tablespoon chopped cilantro if desired. Cook for a final two minutes, stirring often.
- Divide the chicken mixture between two or three tortillas and top with shredded cheese and more chopped cilantro (if desired). Have a salad with your favorite dressing as a side. Drink water, tea, or coffee.

Day 3: Fast day

Breakfast – Skip

Lunch: Asian Chicken Salad

Ingredients:

A boneless, skinless chicken breast

Salad (lettuce or spinach)

Fresh coriander, chopped

Onion

Cucumber

A lime

Brown sugar

Fish sauce

Directions:

- Put the chicken breast in a pot and cover with water. Bring water to a boil and cook chicken for ten minutes. When the chicken is cooked, tear it into shreds using two forks. Combine the salad and the fresh coriander in a bowl. Chop the onion and the cucumber. Mix the onion, cucumber, and chicken and place on top of the salad in the bowl. Juice half of the lime. In a second bowl, mix one tablespoon of fish sauce, the lime juice, and one teaspoon of brown sugar until the sugar dissolves. Pour over the salad.
- Drink water, tea, or coffee.

Dinner: Cherry Tomato Gnocchi

Ingredients:

Gnocchi (1 package)

Cherry tomatoes

Fresh sage

Garlic

Olive oil

Salt

Pepper

Directions:

- Cook the gnocchi according to the instructions on the packaging. Cut ½ cup cherry tomatoes in half and cut one small clove of garlic into thin slices. Heat ½ tablespoon olive oil in a pan. Add the tomatoes and garlic, season with a pinch of salt and pepper, and cook until tomatoes soften. Chop the fresh sage and add all but a pinch to the tomatoes and garlic.
- Top the cooked gnocchi with the tomato, garlic, and sage mixture. Add the final pinch of sage as a garnish.

Day 4: Non-fast day

Breakfast: Soft-Boiled Eggs and Toast

Ingredients:

Eggs

Butter

Whole wheat bread

Directions:

- Heat a couple inches of water in a small saucepan. Once the water is simmering, place two eggs gently in the pan. Simmer for five minutes. Pour off the hot water. For one minute, run cold water over the eggs. Toast and butter two pieces of whole wheat bread. Peel the eggs and spread them on the toast, or cut the toast into strips and dip each strip in the soft-boiled egg.
- Drink water, tea, or coffee.

Lunch: Toasted Margherita Sandwich

Ingredients:

Whole wheat bread

A small tomato

Fresh basil

Fresh mozzarella

Salt

Pepper

Olive oil

Directions:

- Layer a piece of bread with slices of tomato, fresh mozzarella, and fresh basil. Sprinkle with salt and pepper and top with another piece of bread. Drizzle each side of the sandwich with a tablespoon of olive oil. Heat a pan and grill each side of the sandwich until bread is toasted and cheese melts.
- Have an apple as a side. Drink water, tea, or coffee.

Snack: An individual-size Greek yogurt

Dinner: Red Pepper and Halibut Skewers

Ingredients:

Halibut (½ lb)

Red bell pepper

Pesto

White wine vinegar

Salt

Skewers

Orzo

Water

Directions:

- Preheat the oven on the broiler setting and lightly grease a baking pan. Cut the halibut and the red bell pepper into one-inch pieces. Mix three tablespoons of pesto with two tablespoons of white wine vinegar. Pour over the halibut and red bell pepper pieces and let sit for five minutes. Put the halibut and red pepper pieces on the skewers, alternating between fish and pepper. Sprinkle with salt. Place on the greased baking sheet and broil for four minutes. Turn, and broil for another four minutes or until done.

- Prepare orzo according to the directions on the package. Serve as a side to the skewers with butter or additional pesto. Drink water, tea, or coffee.

Day 5: Non-fast day

Breakfast: Bran Muffins

Ingredients:

1 ½ cups wheat flour

¼ cup wheat bran

½ tsp salt

1 tsp baking powder

1 tsp baking soda

2 tablespoons butter, melted

1 cup Greek yogurt

½ cup brown sugar

1 tsp vanilla

1 banana, mashed

1 egg

Directions:

- Preheat the oven to 375 degrees Fahrenheit. Grease a muffin tin. Mix wheat flour, wheat bran, salt, baking powder, and baking soda in one bowl. Combine melted butter, yogurt, brown sugar, vanilla, banana, and egg in a second bowl. Stir flour mixture into yogurt mixture. Bake for twenty-two minutes. This recipe makes twelve muffins. Portion size: two to three muffins.

- Drink water, tea, or coffee.

Lunch: Cream Cheese and Pear Sandwich

Ingredients:

Light cream cheese

A pear

Walnuts

Alfalfa sprouts

Whole wheat bread

Directions:

- Toast two slices of bread and spread each with about one tablespoon of cream cheese. Layer thin slices of pear, finely chopped walnuts, and alfalfa sprouts on one slice of toast. Top with the second slice of toast.
- Have a salad with your favorite dressing as aside. Drink water, coffee, or tea.

Snack: Two oranges

Dinner: Sticky Chicken Thighs

Ingredients:

Two chicken thighs

Olive oil

Salt

Pepper

Onion

Water

Lemon juice

Honey

Couscous

Directions:

- Sprinkle salt and pepper on the chicken thighs and heat ½ tablespoon olive oil in a pan. Set the chicken thighs in the pan and cook for four or five minutes on each side until browned. Remove from the pan and keep warm.

- Add two tablespoons thinly sliced onion to the pan and cook until the onions soften and brown, about two minutes. Add ½ tablespoon lemon juice, one tablespoon water, and ½ tablespoon honey to the onions. Cook for one minute. Set the chicken thighs back into the pan and coat with the onion mixture.

- To make the couscous, heat ½ cup water and a dash of olive oil in a small pot with a tight-fitting lid. When the water boils, pour in ¼ cup couscous, cover, and remove from the heat. Let the pot sit for five minutes until the couscous has absorbed all the water. Fluff with a fork.
- Serve the sticky chicken thighs with couscous and a salad with your favorite dressing. Drink water, tea, or coffee.

Day 6: Fast day

Breakfast – Skip

Lunch: Mediterranean Salad

Ingredients:

Salad (lettuce or spinach)

Sardines in tomato sauce

Capers

Black olives

Olive oil

Red wine vinegar

Directions:

- Place about one cup salad in a bowl. Drain the sardines into a second bowl. Mix the tomato juice from the sardines with the olive oil and red wine vinegar. Chop the olives, combine with the sardines and the capers, and sprinkle over the salad. Top with the tomato, olive oil, and red wine dressing.
- Drink water, tea, or coffee.

Dinner: Avocado Toast with Roast Tomatoes

Ingredients:

Avocado

Tomato

Olive oil

Whole wheat bread

Lemon juice

Chili powder

Spinach

Directions:

- Cut a small tomato into ¼ inch slices. Heat ½ tablespoon of olive oil in a pan and roast the tomatoes until they are soft. Mash one avocado and mix with a pinch of chili powder and one tablespoon lemon juice. Toast the whole wheat bread. Spread the mashed avocado on the bread. Top with the roast tomatoes and a sprinkle of spinach.

Day 7: Non-fast day

Breakfast: Sunny-Side Up Eggs with Muffin Toast

Ingredients:

Olive oil

Eggs

Bran muffins

Butter

Salt

Pepper

Directions:

- Heat olive oil gently in a pan. Crack two eggs into the pan. Cover the pan. Cook about five minutes, or until the yolks are as cooked as you would like. Slice two bran muffins (from Day 5) in half and butter them. Heat a second pan and place the muffin halves butter-side down. Cook until toasted. Salt and pepper the eggs and enjoy with the toasted muffins.

- Drink water, tea, or coffee.

Lunch: Ham Sandwich with Cranberry Chutney

Ingredients:

Whole wheat bread

Mustard

Smoked deli ham

Lettuce or spinach

Cranberry chutney

Directions:

- Spread two slices of bread with mustard. Add a layer of deli ham and a layer of cranberry chutney to one slice of bread. Top with lettuce or spinach and the second slice of bread. For a hot sandwich, toast in a panini grill or on the stove.
- Have an apple as a side. Drink water, coffee, or tea.

Snack: ½ cup dried fruit (apricots, raisins, craisins, dates, blueberries, bananas, etc.)

Dinner: Mustard-Rubbed Salmon Fillet

Ingredients:

One salmon fillet

Mustard

Ground turmeric

Garlic powder

Ground red pepper

Honey

Salt

Spinach

Rice

Water

Directions:

- Preheat the oven on the broiler setting. Line a pan with tinfoil and spray with cooking spray if desired. To prepare the salmon, mix one teaspoon mustard and ½ teaspoon honey with ⅛ teaspoon ground turmeric, a pinch of garlic powder, ⅛ teaspoon ground red pepper, and ⅛ teaspoon salt. Rub the salmon fillet with the mustard mixture and place on the pan. Broil for eight minutes.

- To prepare the rice, boil ⅔ cup salted water in a pot with a tight-fitting lid. Add ⅓ cup rice

407

and reduce heat to low. Simmer for between fifteen and twenty minutes, until all the water is absorbed.

- To prepare the spinach, put one cup of fresh spinach leaves in a steamer or a microwave-safe bowl. Heat the spinach on the stove or in the microwave until just wilted, two or three minutes.
- Serve the salmon with the rice and the spinach as sides. Drink water, tea, or coffee.

Day 8: Training Day

Breakfast – Skip

Lunch: Chicken Stir-Fry with Snow Peas, Broccoli and Mushrooms

Ingredients:

2 (4 oz.) boneless chicken breast

2 cups broccoli florets

1 cup snow peas

1 cup mushrooms – sliced

4 Tbsp. chicken broth

3 tsp. low-sodium soy sauce

2 tsp. sesame oil

1 cup brown rice, steamed

Directions:

- In a large skillet, lightly coat with olive oil or cooking spray and cook chicken over medium heat – about 10 minutes. Remove chicken from pan and stir in the mushrooms, broccoli, and snow peas. Cook vegetables until slightly softened – about 6 minutes. Then return the chicken to the pan and season with sesame oil, soy sauce, chicken broth. Serve with ½ cup brown rice.

Dinner: Lean Pizza

Ingredients:

62 g tortilla bread (2 slices)

20 g tomato pure

65 g cheese (5% fat)

50 g ham

30 g shrimps

20 g mushrooms

40 g tomato

Fresh basil and oregano

Directions:

- Preheat oven to 350 degrees. Prepare the pizza by placing two slices of tortilla bread on a baking sheet. Spread the tomato sauce over the tortilla bread. Then add cheese, ham, shrimp, tomatoes, and mushrooms. Place in oven and bake for 10 minutes. Allow to cool and add fresh basil and oregano. Enjoy!

Day 9: Cardio Day

Breakfast - Skip

Lunch: Chicken & Rice Bowl

Ingredients:

2 oz. chicken breast, grilled & diced

1/3 cup corn

1/3 cup green peas

½ cup brown rice – steamed

Directions:

- Prepare food items according to directions. Combine chicken with corn, green peas, and rice and mix. Enjoy!

Dinner: Lean Turkey Burger

Ingredients:

4 oz. ground lean turkey

2 tbsp. low-sodium salsa

2 tbsp. onion, chopped finely

1 whole-grain hamburger bun

1 cup green beans – steamed

Directions:

- Combine ground turkey, onion and salsa and mix. Form into one large burger patty and frill until cooked. Place patty on bun and serve with green beans on the side.

Day 10: Training Day

Breakfast - Skip

Lunch: Chicken Meatballs

Ingredients:

3 oz. ground lean chicken

1 egg white

1 cup green beans – cooked

½ cup tomato sauce

½ whole-grain pasta – cooked

1 tbsp. bread crumbs

Directions:

- Preheat oven to 375 degrees. Combine the ground chicken with egg white and bread crumbs. Mix well and form into 1-inch meatballs. Place meatballs on a baking sheet and bake for 15 – 20 minutes. Serve meatballs over pasta and tomato sauce with green beans on the side.

Dinner: Grilled Salmon with Steamed Asparagus

Ingredients:

4 oz. Salmon fillet

1 tsp. honey mustard

1/c cup whole-wheat pasta, cooked al dente

Asparagus – steamed

Directions:

- Spread honey mustard for salmon filet. Broil or frill for 12 minutes or until cooked. Serve salmon over pasta with steamed asparagus on the side. Enjoy!

Exercise: Shoulders/Triceps

Rest Between Set 1:30 min

10 Barbell Shoulder Press x 3 reps

10 Dumbbell Arnold Press x 3 reps

8 Close-Grip Bench Press Press x 3 reps

6 Dumbbell Lateral Raise x 3 reps

4 Weighted Tricep Dips x 3 reps

Day 11: Rest Day

Breakfast - Skip

Lunch: Citrus Chicken with Glazed Carrots

Ingredients

4 oz. boneless chicken breast

1 cup carrots – sliced and sliced

2 tbsp. lemon juice

1/2 tbsp. virgin olive oil

2 tsp. honey

½ tsp. paprika

Sea salt and pepper

Directions:

- Preheat oven to 375 degrees. Place chicken breast on a dish, topped with lemon juice, olive oil, sea salt, paprika, and pepper. Place in the oven and bake for 15 – 20 minutes, or until well cooked. While baking, mix the honey glaze with carrots. Serve chicken breasts with glazed honey.

Dinner: Steak with Broccoli

Ingredients:

3 oz. flank or sirloin steak

1 small baked potato

2 tbsp. Dijon mustard

1 cup broccoli – steamed

Lemon juice

Sea salt and pepper

Directions:

- Lightly brush steak with olive oil and sprinkle salt and pepper to taste. Grill steak evenly on both sides for five minutes or until desired doneness. Serve steak along with Dijon mustard, baked potato and lemon-spritzed broccoli.

Day 12: Training Day

Breakfast - Skip

Lunch: Lean Burger

Ingredients:

4 oz. lean ground beef

1 whole wheat English muffin

1 cup mixed greens

½ cup berries

Directions:

- Form ground beef into hamburger patty. Broil or grill the meat patty. Place patty over English muffin and serve with mixed greens and berries on the side.

Dinner: Whole Wheat Pasta with Feta Cheese and Veggies

Ingredients:

¾ cup pasta – whole wheat

1/3 cup feta cheese

1 cup mixed veggies

Directions:

- Cook pasta according to package. Top pasta with crumbled feta cheese and mixed vegetables.

Exercise: Back Day

Rest Between Set 1:30 min

10 Wide-grip pull ups x 3 reps

8 Narrow Grin chinup x 3 reps

6 Bent Over Barbbell Row x 3 reps

6 Bent Over Barbbell Row x 3 reps

4Barbbell Deadlift x 3 reps

Day 13: Cardio Day

Breakfast - Skip

Lunch: Baked Cod with Steamed Vegetable Medley

Ingredients:

4 oz. Cod filet

2 tbsp. bread crumbs

1 tsp. Olive oil

Salt and pepper

1 cup mixed vegetables – steamed

Directions:

- Preheat oven to 375 degrees. Coat cod fillet with salt, pepper, olive oil and bread crumbs. Place on baking sheet and bake for 12-15 minutes until flakey results. Serve cod with 1 cup of steamed vegetables on the side.

Dinner: Dinner Omelet

Ingredients:

1 egg – whole

2 egg whites

1 slice whole-wheat bread

1 cup baby spinach

¼ cup feta cheese

Directions:

- In a skillet, lightly coat with cooking spray. Mix egg, egg whites, spinach, and feta cheese together until well-combined. Cook mixture for 3 minutes or until well cooked. Serve omelet with whole-wheat bread.

Day 14: Rest Day

Breakfast - Skip

Lunch: Roast Beef Wrap

Ingredients:

4 oz. lean roast beef –sliced

2 slices avocado

1 small tomato- sliced

1 whole-grain tortilla

1 cup mixed berries – fresh or frozen

Directions:

- Place tortilla on plate. Add the beef slices, avocado, and tomato in tortilla and roll. Serve with mixed berries on the side. Enjoy!

Dinner: Rotisserie Chicken Dish

Ingredients:

4 oz. Rotisserie chicken breast

1 tsp. olive oil

1 tsp. lemon juice

1 cup mixed greens

1 granny smith apple – chopped

Directions:

- Serve chicken with mixed green salad with olive oil and lemon juice. Add sliced apple as dessert.

Day 15: Training Day

Breakfast - Skip

Lunch: Shrimp Cocktail Platter

Ingredients:

4 oz. shrimp – boiled and cooled

1 whole wheat dinner roll

1 cup mixed vegetables

2 tbsp. cocktail sauce

Fresh lemon

Directions:

- Serve prepared shrimp with cocktail sauce and lemon. Enjoy dinner and mixed vegetables on the side.

Dinner: Protein Pizza Tortilla

Ingredients:

1 whole-grain tortilla

2 oz. grilled chicken- sliced

¼ cup tomato sauce

¼ mozzarella cheese –skimmed

1 cup broccoli – steamed

Directions:

- Preheat oven to 350 degrees. Add tomato sauce, mozzarella cheese, and chicken to the tortilla. Bake for 10 minutes and serve with steamed broccoli on the side.

Day 16: Cardio

Breakfast - Skip

Lunch: Sashimi

Ingredients:

3 oz. fresh sashimi

½ cup brown rice – cooked

2 tbsp. Asian ginger dressing

Mixed green salad

Directions:

- Slice sashimi into 6 pieces. Add a side of rice and mixed green salad topped with Asian dressing.

Dinner: Turkey Chili

Ingredients:

1 cup turkey chili – homemade or store bought

2 egg whites – hard boiled

2 tbsp. red wine vinegar

1 tsp. olive oil

1 cup mixed green salad

Directions:

- Serve chili with 2 hard-boiled egg whites and a side of mixed green salad with oil and vinegar.

Day 17: Training

Breakfast - Skip

Lunch: Turkey Lettuce Wrap with Bean Salad

Ingredients:

2 oz. deli turkey breast slices

1 tbsp. Russian dressing

1 tomato – sliced

Large lettuce leaves

¼ cup chickpeas

¼ cup tomato – chopped

¼ cup celery – chopped

¼ cup kidney beans

1 tsp. virgin olive oil

Lemon juice

Salt and pepper

Directions:

- Prepare lettuce leaves with turkey, sliced tomato and Russian dressing in a wrap. Serve lettuce wrap with mixed bean salad.

Dinner: Tuna-Tomato Salad

Ingredients:

4 oz. water-packed tuna can

1 large tomato – hallowed, remove seeds

3 pcs whole-grain toast

¼ cup celery – chopped

¼ cup red onion – chopped

1 tbsp. low-fat mayonnaise

1 tsp. Dijon mustard

Directions:

- Combine Tuna, onion, celery, mayonnaise, and mustard and mix. Place mixture into hollowed tomato. Serve with toast.

Day 18: Rest Day

Breakfast - Skip

Lunch: Cold Cut Platter

Makes one serving; 289 calories, 12g fat, 27g protein, and 20 carbs per serving.

Ingredients:

2 oz. sliced ham

2 oz. deli turkey breast

1 oz. low-fat Swiss cheese – sliced thinly

1 ripe tomato – sliced

Whole-grain crackers – 100 calories worth

Directions:

- Prepare your own cracker sandwiches with the ingredients provided.

Dinner: Turkey Chili

Makes one serving; 310 calories, 10g fat, 23g protein, 30g carbs per serving.

Ingredients:

1 cup chili – turkey or veggie

2 egg whites – hard boiled

Red wine vinegar

1 tsp. olive oil

Mixed greens

Directions:

- Prepare chili as directed. Serve chili with 2 hard-boiled eggs with oil and vinegar over a mixed green salad.

Day 19: Training Day

Breakfast - Skip

Lunch: Protein Nut Butter and Jelly Sandwich

Ingredients:

1 slice whole-grain bread slice

1 tbsp. fruit preserves

1 tbsp. nut butter – peanut or almond

½ cup cottage cheese

Directions:

- Cut bread slice in half. Add nut butter and preserves and combine. Serve with cottage cheese on the side.

Dinner: Cold Meat Platter

Ingredients:

2 oz. turkey breast – sliced

1 oz. low-fat Swiss cheese- sliced

2 oz. ham – sliced

1 tomato – sliced

Whole-grain crackers – 100 calories worth

Directions:

- Create your mini cracker sandwiches with the included ingredients.

Exercise: Back

Rest Between Set 1:30 min

4 Barbell Deadlift x 4 reps

6 Chin Up x 4 reps

10 Close Grip Chin Up x 10 reps

Day 20: Cardio Day

Breakfast - Skip

Lunch: Sashimi

Ingredients:

3 oz. sashimi – 6 pcs

½ cup brown rice – steamed

2 tbsp. Asian ginger dressing

1 cup mixed green salad

Directions:

- Enjoy cut sashimi with a side of brown rice and mixed green salad topped with Asian dressing to complete the set.

Dinner: Whole Wheat Pasta with Feta and Vegetables

Ingredients:

1 cup mixed steamed vegetables

1/3 cup feta cheese

¾ cup whole-wheat pasta

Directions:

- Add mixed steam vegetables and feta cheese to whole-wheat pasta for a light dinner dish. Enjoy!

Day 21: Rest Day

Breakfast - Skip

Lunch: Chicken Ranch Wrap

Ingredients:

1 whole-grain tortilla slice

1 tomato – slice

2 slices lettuce

Celery sticks – handful

1 tbsp. ranch dressing

Directions:

- Fill tortilla wrap with chicken breast, tomato, lettuce, and top with ranch dressing. Serve with celery sticks on the side.

Dinner: Salmon Nicoise

Ingredients:

3 oz. salmon fillet

5 black olives

2 cups mixed green salad

1 cup green beans

1 small red potato – boiled

Lemon juice

Salt and pepper

Directions:

- Cook Salmon as desired. Add two cups of mixed greens with beans, olives, and potato.

Season with freshly squeezed lemon juice salt and pepper.

Day 22: Cardio Day

Breakfast - Skip

Lunch: Stuffed Peppers Provençale

Ingredients

2 Red Bell Peppers

4 Artichoke Hearts (tinned, not oil, 88g)

4 Cherry Tomatoes (45g)

4 Black Olives, drained (10g)

2 Anchovy Fillets, rinsed and drained (8g)

2 tbsp Fresh Basil, cut into strips

2 sprays Frylight Olive Oil Spray

Pinch Ground Black Pepper

Pinch Sea (Kosher) Salt

Directions

- Preheat the oven to 180C fan, 375F, Gas Mark 6.
- Start by rinsing well all the canned foods (artichoke hearts, olives, anchovy fillets) to

remove canning brine and salt, and then pat dry on kitchen towel.

- With a sharp kitchen knife, cut each pepper in half through the stalk. Remove the pith and seeds and discard but keep the stalk in place as it will help keep the peppers in shape when cooking. Transfer the halves, cut sides up, into a roasting tin.
- Cut in half the artichoke hearts, olives and tomatoes and distribute evenly between the 4 pepper halves. Chop up the anchovy fillets and pop them into gaps in the stuffed peppers. Finally, chiffonade (cut into thin strips) the basil leaves, scatter over the stuffed peppers and spritz them with 2 sprays of Frylight Olive Oil Spray.
- Cover the roasting tin loosely with tin foil and bake in the oven for 25 mins.
- The peppers can be served immediately hot from the oven, or allowed to cool and served at room temperature for a packed lunch.

Dinner: Fettuccine Chicken Alfredo

Ingredients:

Alfredo Sauce

2 cloves garlic

2 tablespoons of butter

1/2 cup of heavy cream

4 tablespoons of grated parmesan

1/2 teaspoon of dried basil

Chicken and noodles

1 tablespoon of olive oil

2 chicken thighs

Miracle Noodle fettuccine noodles 1 bag

Salt and pepper

Directions:

- Put some chopped garlic with butter in the skillet over low heat for around 2 minutes. Add the heavy cream and allow it to heat for 2 additional minutes.
- Add the parmesan, 1 tablespoon at a time while stirring. Add the seasoning and the dried basil and let them cook for 4 minutes on low heat until they start thickening. Now, you have your alfredo sauce.
- Add some oil to another pan over medium heat and fry your chicken thighs for about 8 minutes. Take them off the heat and shred them.
- Boil some clean miracle noodles for about 3 minutes.

431

- Put the noodles in the pan with the chicken, add the alfredo sauce and mix for 3 minutes over medium heat.
- Serve and enjoy!

Day 23: Training Day

Breakfast - Skip

Lunch: Grilled Ruben Sandwich

Ingredients

28g (1 oz) thinly sliced Pastrami

15g (1 tbsp) 3% Fat Soft Cheese

10g (1½ tbsp) grated 50% Reduced Fat Mature Cheddar Cheese

2 tbsp Sauerkraut, rinsed and drained

1 tsp Tomato ketchup

1 Dill Pickle, rinsed and drained, sliced

1 Soft Brown Sandwich Thin

Directions

- Preheat the grill or health grill. Rinse and drain the pickle and sauerkraut to remove excess salt. Mix together the ketchup and soft cheese, divide the sandwich thin and spread with the mixture. Onto one of the sandwich thin halves, layer up the sauerkraut, pastrami, dill pickle slices and grated cheese. Top with the remaining sandwich thin half and secure with a cocktail stick.

- Cook the sandwiches for 2-3 minutes in a health grill or cook for 2 minutes each side under a cooker grill.

Dinner: Spicy Crockpot Double Beef Stew

Ingredients

1.5lbs Beef Stew

2 14.5oz cans chili-ready diced tomatoes (organic)

1 tbsp. chili mix (pre-packaged or one you made yourself)

1 cup beef broth

2 tsp hot sauce

1 tbsp. Worcestershire sauce

salt (to taste)

Directions

- Turn your crockpot on to high, add all the ingredients and mix.
- Cook for about 6 hours on high.

- Break up the meat with a fork and pull apart within the crockpot.
- Add salt to taste.
- Cook for 2 hours on low.

Day 24: Rest Day

Breakfast - Skip

Lunch: Low-Carbohydrate Pizza

Ingredients:

¾ cup of mozzarella

½ cup of Marinara sauce

4 slices of pepperoni

½ tsp of basil

½ tsp of oregano

Directions:

- Put ½ of your mozzarella cheese into a frying pan, and allow it to heat and melt and it will caramelize too. When it's reasonably dark in colour, use a spatula to lift the disk of cheese from out of the frying pan. This will be the base for your pizza.

- Next pour over the marina sauce making sure it covers all your cheese base and goes right to the edges.
- Place the remaining mozzarella on top of the pizza, and the pepperoni slices too.
- Sprinkle on the seasoning of basil and oregano.
- Heat under a grill until the mozzarella on top of the pizza has melted.

Dinner: Goat-Cheese, Avocado and Bacon Salad

Ingredients:

Goat cheese - 230 g

Bacon- 230 g

Avocados - 2 pcs

Walnuts - 115 g

Arugula lettuce - 115 g

Dressing

Fresh juice of ½ lemon

Homemade mayonnaise - 120 g

Olive oil - 120 g

Double cream - 50 g

Directions:

- Before you start cooking this wonderful salad, switch on the oven and preheat it to 200°C . Place greaseproof paper in a shallow round cake pan.
- Cut cheese into round slices (about 25 mm) and place in your round cake pan. Bake until golden crust.
- Take bacon, slice it and fry until crispy.
- Take an avocado wash it and dry with a paper towel, cut into small blocks.
- Place arugula lettuce on the plate. On top of the leaves put the avocado cubs, add the fried crispy bacon and round slices of fried goat cheese. Sprinkle with crushed walnuts.
- Blend ingredients for a salad flavoring: freshly squeezed lemon juice, 120 g of olive oil, mayonnaise - 120 g and double cream - 50 g. Put a teaspoon of fresh herbs.
- Salt and pepper to taste.

Day 25: Cardio Day

Breakfast - Skip

Lunch: Sweet Chilli Prawn Stir Fry

Ingredients:

60g (2/3 Cup) Chinese Leaf /Nappa Cabbage, chopped

1 Medium Carrot (60g)

½ Red Bell Pepper

50g (1/3 Cup) Frozen podded Soya Edamame Beans

60g (½ Cup) Beansprouts (Mung)

100g (1 Cup) Chestnut (Baby Portabella) Mushrooms

60g (½ Cup) Mange Tout (Snow Peas

60g (½ Cup) Baby Corn

2 tbsp Thai Sweet Chilli Sauce

100g (2/3 Cup) Cooked King Prawn/Shrimp

Pinch Sea (Kosher) Salt

1 Garlic Clove

2 sprays Frylight Olive Oil Spray

Directions:

- Cut the carrot and bell pepper into strips. Clean the mushrooms and slice. Halve the mange tout and baby corn.
- Heat up a wok over a medium heat and spritz twice with Frylight olive oil spray. Start stir frying the peppers, mushrooms, carrot and baby corn. After 3 mins, add in the remaining vegetables and continue stir frying for another 3 mins.
- Add the edamame beans and prawns and continue to cook until the beans have fully defrosted and the prawns have warmed through completely. Remove from heat and stir through the Thai sweet chilli sauce.
- Season with salt and serve.

Dinner: Basil and Parmesan Stuffed Chicken Breasts:

Ingredients:

4 Chicken Breasts, boneless and skinless

1 Cup Parmesan Cheese, shredded or grated

1/4 Cup Cream Cheese, full fat

1/4 Cup Fresh Basil, chopped

1 Garlic Clove, minced

2 TBSP Coconut Oil (or extra virgin olive oil)

1/8 TSP Pink Himalayan Salt

1/8 TSP Black Pepper, fresh ground

Directions:

- In a small saucepan over low heat, melt together: parmesan cheese, cream cheese, basil, garlic, pink Himalayan salt, and black pepper.
- While the above mixture heats, cut pockets into each chicken breast. Cut this pocket into the thick side so it cooks evenly and doesn't fall apart during the cooking process.
- Using all except about 1/4 cup of the filling, stuff each chicken breast evenly. Using two tooth picks per piece of chicken, seal the opened side of the chicken breast to keep the filling from falling out during cooking process.
- In a medium frying pan, melt the oil until its hot and then cook the chicken for about 5 minutes on each side. Make sure each side is browned, and cooked evenly through.
- After the chicken is cooked on either side, cover them with the remaining cheese filling and cover the frying pan with a lid. Let them continue to cook until the cheese melts, and then serve hot.

Day 26: Rest Day

Breakfast - Skip

Lunch: Mung Beans & Spinach Soup

Ingredients:

2 1/2 cups cooked Sprouted Mung Beans

3 cups fresh baby spinach

1 tbs. oil

3 cloves garlic, minced

1 medium onion, sliced

1 small tomatoes, diced

Juice of 1 lime

Salt to taste

2 cups water

Directions:

- In your Instant Pot sauté garlic and onions in olive oil for two minutes stirring frequently. Add salt to taste.
- Place all remaining ingredient in the Instant Pot.
- Cover lid and set for Bean for 15 minutes.
- Allow pressure to come down naturally when done. Stir for a few minutes until all ingredients are cooked well.

- Adjust salt to taste. Turn off your Instant Pot.
- Serve hot.

Dinner: Pasta Carbonara

Ingredients:

3 servings of Slim Pasta

5 oz. bacon

2 egg yolks

1 whole egg

1 tbsp. heavy cream

1/3 cup grated parmesan

3 tbsp. chopped basil

Black pepper to taste

Directions:

- Begin by preparing your pasta according to the directions on the packet.
- Continue by cutting your bacon in to cubes and cook it in a deep skillet until you get a crispy bacon. Once cooked, keep just 1/3 of your bacon grease and set the bacon aside on a small plate.
- Next, throw your egg, parmesan cheese, and egg yolks in to your saved bacon grease and

mix your ingredients together until they are well combined.

- Finally, add your Slim Pasta in to the bacon grease mixture and cook on high until your pasta is a little crispy.
- Remove your crispy pasta mixture from the heat and mix everything together in your pan. Separate in to 3 servings and if desired season with black pepper before serving.

Day 27: Cardio Day

Breakfast - Skip

Lunch: Tuna 'Mayo' Sandwich

Ingredients:

60g (2 oz) No-drain, pole and line caught Tuna in Brine

20g (1 tbsp + 1 tsp) 3% Fat Soft Cheese

20g (½ Cup) Fresh Watercress

Whole-wheat Sandwich Thin

Directions:

- Flake the tuna fish into a bowl and combine with the cheese. Open the sandwich thin and fill with tuna mix and watercress. Sandwich thin together and serve.

Day 28: Training Day

Breakfast - Skip

Lunch: Cauliflower Gratin (V)

Ingredients:

300g (3 Cups) Cauliflower Florets

120mls (½ Cup) Semi-Skimmed (Reduced Fat) Milk

20g (3 tbsp) grated 50% Reduced Fat Mature Cheddar Cheese

7g (1 tbsp) finely grated Fresh Parmesan Cheese

½ tsp Dry Mustard Powder

1 tbsp Cornflour/Cornstarch

Pinch Ground Black Pepper

Pinch Sea (Kosher) Salt

Directions:

- Preheat the oven to 180C fan, 375F, Gas Mark 6.
- Lightly steam the cauliflower florets for 5 mins, then transfer to an ovenproof dish.

- Meanwhile, in a small bowl, slacken (dissolve) the cornflour (cornstarch) with a little of the cold milk. Heat the rest of the milk until just before simmering, stir the dissolved cornstarch again to make sure that it is still fully dissolved then quickly whisk the mixture into the hot milk. Continue whisking until the sauce thickens, then allow to simmer gentle for 1 min. Whisk in the mustard powder and the grated cheeses. Stir until cheese has melted and season with salt and pepper to taste.
- Pour over the cauliflower florets and bake in the oven until golden brown.

Dinner: Baked Salmon

Ingredients:

2 (6-ounce) salmon fillets

1 tablespoon fresh parsley, chopped

1 tablespoon lemon juice

1 teaspoon black pepper, ground

1 teaspoon salt

1 teaspoon dried basil

6 tablespoons light olive oil

2 cloves garlic, minced

Directions:

- Mix parsley, lemon juice, pepper, salt, basil, olive oil and garlic to prepare the marinade.
- Put the salmon filets into a separate medium glass baking dish and cover the filets with the marinade. Allow to marinate for about 1 hour in the fridge.
- Preheat the oven to 375 degrees F, then put the fillets on aluminum foil, and cover the filets with more marinade.
- Put the filets on the foil into the glass baking dish and bake in the preheated oven for around 35 minutes. When ready, the salmon should easily flake.

Day 29: Rest Day

Breakfast - Skip

Lunch: Mocha Truffles

Ingredients:

1 Cup Unsalted Butter, softened

3-4 Tablespoons of Very Strong Coffee

2 Tablespoons of Cacao Powder

2 Tablespoons Sukrin Gold, or sweetener of your choice

½ Teaspoon of Ground Cinnamon

½ Teaspoon of Vanilla Powder

Direction:

- In a bowl, combine butter with the rest of the ingredients. Use a fork to mix it well together.
- Make little truffles either using your hands or two teaspoons. Place them on a plate covered with parchment paper and put them in the freezer or fridge.

Dinner: Zucchini & Bacon Stir-Fry

Ingredients:

4 slices bacon, chopped

1 ounce onion, chopped, 1/4 cup

2 medium zucchini, cut in half moons, 12 ounces

Salt and pepper, to taste

2 eggs, fried in 1 tablespoon butter

Directions:

- In a medium skillet, fry the bacon until it starts to brown and render its fat. Add the onion and zucchini.

- Cook and stir over medium-high heat until the zucchini is tender and caramelized and the bacon is cooked completely.
- Season to taste with salt and pepper while cooking. Transfer the zucchini mixture to a serving plate and keep warm.
- In the same skillet, fry two eggs in butter. Serve the eggs over the zucchini mixture.

Day 30: Cardio Day

Breakfast - Skip

Lunch: Tuna Salad

Ingredients:

1 tablespoon extra-virgin olive oil

1 tablespoon fresh lemon juice

1 medium bunch chives or spring onions

2 tablespoons mayonnaise

2 organic eggs, hard-boiled

140g canned tuna, drained

1 small head lettuce, Little Gem or Romaine

Salt such as pink Himalayan

Directions:

- Wash and drain the lettuce leaves and place them in a serving bowl. Add drained, shredded tuna on top of the lettuce.
- Top with mayo, hard-boiled eggs, and the chopped spring onions.
- Drizzle with olive oil, and serve.

Dinner: Sausage and Pepper Soup

Ingredients:

32 oz. pork sausage

¾ teaspoon kosher salt

1 teaspoon Italian seasoning

1 teaspoon garlic powder

1 tablespoon cumin

1 tablespoon chili powder

1 teaspoon onion powder

4 cups beef stock

1 can tomatoes with jalapeños

1 medium green bell pepper

10 oz. raw spinach

1 tablespoon olive oil

Directions:

- In a large pot, heat olive oil and then add sausage to the pot.
- After the sausage sears, mix it and let it cook for some time. Meanwhile, slice the bell pepper and then add it to the pot; season with pepper and salt.
- Add jalapeños and tomatoes and stir. Add spinach on top and cover with lid.
- Cook for about 6-7 minutes and allow the spinach to wilt. As the this cooks, prepare the beef stock and the spices.
- Mix the spinach with the sausage, and add spices. Then add the beef stock and mix well.
- Cover and cook for 30 minutes over medium-low heat. Once done, remove the lid and allow to simmer for 15 minutes.

Do's And Don'ts of Intermittent Fasting For Women

Do keep tabs on your hormone health.

The biggest risk women have with intermittent fasting is with their hormones. Our hormones play a very delicate balancing act on a repeated 28-day cycle (on average). Sometimes the slightest change in our diet, health, mindset, environment, toxin exposure, or stress-level can cause hormonal imbalance to occur leading to further health issues down the road. If not done properly, intermittent fasting could easily become one of these triggers for hormonal imbalance because of the stress it can cause on your body.

It's not only the sex hormones that can be affected. Cortisol and thyroid hormones are also very important to monitor, especially if you have had past issues with thyroid disorders or adrenal fatigue.

Following the steps listed below will help tremendously in keeping your hormones balanced and stress level regulated. It is also very important to check on the state of your hormones before you even begin. If you are already dealing with a hormonal imbalance of any kind, addressing that issue will need to precede the intermittent fasting plan. The best way to do this is to test both your daily cortisol rhythm and your monthly hormonal cycle with a salivary collection.

Don't diet.

Ok, are you ready for the biggest reason why intermittent fasting DOESN'T work for women? Because we also try to diet at the same time! This is not the concept behind intermittent fasting and will ultimately either lead to bingeing, failure, or health and hormonal issues. During the period of time you are eating, you need to EAT. Eat a lot of really nutrient-dense, calorically-dense foods in that timeframe and do not try to be in a huge calorie deficit. This won't work. I like to think of intermittent fasting as a better, safer, smarter option to restricting calories. But, definitely never do both.

Do focus on fats.

In order to make sure you're not going into too big of a calorie deficit, your diet will need to consist primarily of healthy, nutrient-dense fats. These include fat from properly raised animals, unsweetened coconut and coconut oil, nuts and nut butters, pasture-raised butter or ghee, eggs, avocado and avocado oil, olives and olive oil, and grass-fed dairy products. When these foods become staples, you can rest assured that you will be getting enough nutrients and calories in your day prior to fasting.

Not only that, but switching to a high-fat diet will also ensure your fasting periods are stress-free, safe, and comfortable. With the reduction of carbohydrates and inclusion of a large amount of fat, your blood sugar will become extremely stable. Instead of being a rollercoaster (which is what happens to our blood sugar when we have excess carbohydrates in our diet), it will be more like small waves. When our bodies are on the rollercoaster route, there will be a dip in blood sugar a few hours after your last meal which brings on feelings of hunger. When no glucose is provided by way of a meal, cortisol – our stress hormone – will come to the rescue. So, now you're hungry, you're still fasting for another 5 hours, and your body senses a stressful event. Not good!

However, when you take a high-fat diet approach and become fat-adapted, that dip in blood sugar doesn't happen and the stressor isn't there because your body no longer relies on only glucose for energy. Your body has learned to run on fats – both dietary and stored body fat – instead of just waiting for the next meal. Now, not only are you not having feelings of hunger, but you're eliminating the stressful event! And, as we discussed above, the reason why intermittent fasting can be hard for women is because of the hormonal imbalance that can develop from the stress and cortisol response. Just by eating high-fat and plenty of food, we have eliminated that stressor!

Don't workout intensely.

At least for the first week or two until you know how intermittent will affect you. Once your body becomes adapted to this change, chances are workouts will actually feel better in the fasted state and you will begin to see improvements in your workouts. But, first you need to eliminate all added stressors while your body adapts and gets used to this new energy source (fat). Taking walks in nature or a really great yoga class will be the best way to get movement in during this transition time. After that, begin incorporating short HIIT sessions like jumping rope, sprinting, or heavy lifts in the gym and see how you feel. Remember, the end goal is to keep the stress level in the body at an all time low, thereby keeping your hormones in balance. Working out too intensely while your body is shifting energy sources will likely cause stress.

Don't make fat loss your main goal.

There are many success stories out there of people who have had complete body composition changes just by incorporating intermittent fasting. And it's true. It is a great tool for losing weight, getting leaner, and decreasing body fat. BUT, I don't think any female should do it just for that purpose. This is not the next way to obsess about your body and try to manipulate its size with food.

This is a therapeutic diet with amazing health benefits and should be viewed as such. Find a deeper purpose behind your dietary changes. Do you have brain fog or trouble concentrating? Intermittent fasting is great for brain health. Want to age well and live longer? Intermittent fasting has been shown to prolong lifespan and slow down the aging process.

Need to get your blood lipids and cardiovascular markers in check? Intermittent fasting can bring those markers back in range without the use of medication.

Do start slow.

Intermittent fasting isn't something you need to dive into all or nothing for it to be effective. In fact, women may have better luck with easing their way into it. Spend 3-4 weeks becoming fat-adapted with a high fat diet first. Then, add in an intermittent fasting schedule a few days per week. For instance, try doing a 16/8 fast on Monday's and Thursday's and see how that feels. If you enjoy it, add in more days as you feel comfortable.

Don't continue if you feel bad.

This should go without saying, but obviously if you are feeling weak, tired, dizzy, or just don't like it, then don't do it! This is not something that will feel right for everyone, so pay attention, listen to your body, and always do what's right for you.

Do enlist the support of a professional.

As with any advice I give, I always recommend seeking the help of a professional to guide you through the changes you wish to make and support you along the way. This will make it easier to acknowledge what is right for YOU instead of just guessing. If you would like help in determining your individualized plan based on the state of your hormones, contact me for a free 15-minute case review.

The 30-Day Plan – Physical Health Benefits

"A little starvation can really do more for the average sick man than can the best medicines and the best doctors" - Mark Twain

In this section, we look in further detail at the clinically proven health benefits of the 30-day plan.

We'll show that Mark Twain was right all those years ago, and that you can reap the benefits without starving yourself (Twain wasn't known for his sensitive use of language, this is the guy who once threatened to dig up Jane Austen and beat her back to death with her own shinbone).

Insulin, Glycogen and Fat Burning

As covered under the science, the primary benefit of IF and our 30-day plan for the vast majority will be the decreased period of INSULTION PRODUCTION in the body, driving a virtuous cycle of increased body fat burning.

In his bestselling IF text Eat Stop Eat, Brad Pilon showed that the amount of stored fat released for oxidation (burning) through the lipolysis process increased by over 50% after only 24 hours of fasting. We'll be getting seven such hits in our 30 days, and the benefits will be dramatic.

Weight Loss

The first think everyone thinks of when anything to do with dieting is mentioned. Due to your decreased calorific intake (around 30% for our plan remember), your body will have the necessary conditions to not only stop weight gain, but also to lose weight. Research has shown that any time we fast for a significant period (>18 hours), we lose two to three pounds in weight.

How much you lose will depend upon a lot of factors, including your metabolic rate (which drives your normal weight gain/loss profile), current weight, your diet and how active you are. As you become familiar with the 30-day regime you will be able to monitor how it is impacting on your body and tweak your food intake and level of exercise to optimize it for you. As we've said, weight loss is not the primary objective for most people who subscribe to the plan, and, particularly if you are fit and healthy, it's possible to reap the benefits without losing a single pound and maintaining your muscle mass – more on that later.

Hormonal Benefits

As your body burns off more fat reserves several secondary processes are invoked or optimized which in turn derive additional benefits for us, particularly at the hormonal level.

Adrenaline

Adrenaline and noradrenalin (also known as epinephrine and norepinephrine) are the body's fight or flight hormones, i.e. in times of stress they increase the blood flow and the oxygen getting to the muscles, essentially increasing your capacity to deal with the situation by fighting or by running away. Physical symptoms are a thumping heart rate and sweating, and mental alertness and focus is increased. Mentally, ALERTNESS and FOCUS increases.

It has been shown that all IF programs serve to increase adrenaline levels, because the body is already in a heightened state of fat burning and not simply adding to its fat reserves. The benefits of this response in terms of energy and productivity levels are apparent, however care does need to be taken in

461

controlling the levels released, which we will explore further below.

Growth Hormone

Human Growth Hormone (HGH) is produced the pituitary gland, not only for children (for whom it is essential), but in all of us. HGH is then released into the bloodstream, only momentarily, before it is sent to the liver for metabolism into several blood factors, most notably Insulin-Like-Growth-Factor (IGFI).

Studies have shown that HGH can increase exponentially following fasting – in one extreme example a man undertaking a forty day fast for religious purposes was found to have 1,250% in growth hormone by the end of the period!

But, I hear you ask, surely that means more IGFI, and didn't we learn in the science bit that insulin is the bad stuff that increases diabetes and drives fat and sugar and all of that? Isn't insulin kryptonite for the dieter? Well YES, but the key thing is in the short release time which allows the body to build resistance to the IGFI while deriving the benefits from HGH.

And those benefits are well documented – synthetic HGH is banned in athletes as a performance enhancing drug for very good reason - it increases blood glucose by driving more fat burning and greatly increases not only energy levels but also muscle mass, therefore conferring an unfair advantage.

There are no rules against naturally increasing your own HGH levels of course, and it's not just elite athletes and bodybuilders who can feel the benefits. A known (and positive) side-effect of increasing lean body mass and loss of fat is thicker and tighter skin – or in other words – ANTI-AGEING. So, you can see how there are benefits for everyone.

Suppressed Hunger

For a lot of people the biggest obstacle to taking on any dietary program (and particularly any that involve the word 'fasting'), is the thought of feeling hungry for most of the time. Nobody wants to go through their day with nagging hunger pangs following them around – hunger can decrease mood, concentration, ability to be productive, and general sense of wellbeing.

Well the good news is that IF should not make you hungry!

There is a lot of heavy science behind what makes us hungry, mostly driven by the balance of hormones including our old friends (insulin, norepinephrine and glucagon) and our bodies' response to fluctuating levels of these. Without getting further into the chemistry, it's an established fact that hunger peaks four to five hours following a meal, only for the feeling to then subside. The good news is that we can override the initial impulse to respond to our hungers pangs (as I write this my stomach is rumbling, but I don't actually feel hungry, so I'm not going to have that snack), and do this after just a couple of days of sticking to our plan.

Essentially we are learning the difference between physical hunger (with tiredness, weakness, irritability and all of that), and psychological hunger (a learned response to our hunger pangs formed out of habit). All it takes is a little perseverance, particularly in the early days. Once you've broken through the envelope, like an airliner emerging from the clouds into brilliant sunshine, you will see a better clearer world driven by the optimized processes in your body; you will have more energy, be more productive, and feel better!

Lower Cholesterol

Alongside high blood pressure and anxiety and depression, high cholesterol is possibly the most widely medicated for condition at a population level.

Hundreds of millions of people worldwide are on long term medication to lower their cholesterol. At one level this makes sense – high cholesterol is a known risk factor for heart attack and stroke, and it can be regulated pharmacologically.

However, this approach is a classic example of filling the bucket and not fixing the roof. Whereas a long-term prescription for cholesterol medication may help control this risk factor, it is doing it unilaterally, with no wider benefit for the patient's health and wellbeing.

Why not assume all the benefits of lower cholesterol while also piling on the associated benefits of a better diet, lifestyle and feeling of wellbeing? And do so without the risks associated with any long-term medication – a decade or so back Pfizer pumped billions into a cholesterol management drug it called torcetrapib, designed to reduce heart attacks – in this instance by increasing the levels of "good" cholesterol (HDL) in the body. The results were staggering, staggeringly bad. Death

rates of those in the study increased by a quarter -
that's dozens of real people dying as they placed their
trust in an experimental drug based on seemingly
sound science.

Even if your medication doesn't have a
weapons-grade killing capability at the population
level, you still don't know what effect it is having on
you and it may also provide a false sense of security
that increases other risk factors in your lifestyle. The
good news is that cholesterol levels can be managed,
and the ratios between "good" and "bad" optimized
simply by embarking on an IF programme.

Inflammation

Inflammation is defined by the Farlex
medical dictionary as "A localized protective
response elicited by injury or destruction of tissues,
which serves to destroy, dilute, or wall off both the
injurious agent and the injured tissue." Causes of
inflammation include physical injury, exposure to

extremes of heat or cold, infectious agents such as viruses and bacteria, and exposure to x-rays and other radioactive sources.

It is considered that almost every chronic disease is caused ultimately by INFLAMMATION, and one of the most powerful factors in increasing the likelihood of an inflammatory response to one of these triggers is - yes you've guessed it - OBESITY. Recent studies have shown that fasting induces a strong anti-inflammatory effect on the body, improving not only immune function but the nervous system in general. Once again we have a non-chemical, rapidly working and proven tool right in front of us to improve our levels of health and wellbeing.

Book 7: Intermittent Fasting

The Unstoppable Intermittent Fasting Beginners Guide to Lose 3 Pounds of Fat a Week, Build Muscle, Stay Lean and Feel Healthier.

By

Beatrice Anahata

Introduction

When it comes to intermittent fasting, most people tend to think of fat loss. Believe it or not, intermittent fasting can also be an effective nutrition strategy for building muscle. Recall some of the benefits I mentioned earlier about fasting—specifically increased growth hormone and increased efficiency using fat for fuel.

The additional growth hormone will help you build more muscle, and you'll be less likely to store fat while you pack on muscle. So then what's the difference between fasting for fat loss and fasting to build muscle? The answer lies in a number of calories you need to eat. The caloric deficit is king for fat loss, and the caloric surplus is king for building muscle.

This means you must eat more calories than you burn off if you want to build muscle. Imagine you're an architect building a 2,600 square foot house. You'll need a certain number of bricks—say

6,000 for example—to build that house. If you don't have 6,000 bricks, then you'll have to downgrade the size of the house you're building.

Your muscles work the same way. If you want to build muscle, you must provide your body with enough of the raw materials (i.e. calories you get from food) necessary for it to happen. If you don't, then you'll be in the same boat as an architect without enough bricks. How many calories do you need to build muscle?

Use this simple equation:

Bodyweight in pounds x16=Daily caloric intake

Using myself as an example:

Bodyweight-195x16=3,120 calories

This means that I need to eat 3,120 calories every day to start gaining weight. One common complaint from guys is that they're a "hard gainer" or that they have a lightning fast metabolism. It doesn't matter how much they eat; they can't seem to gain any weight. The issue isn't that you're a hard gainer, it's the fact that you're not measuring how much you're eating.

You might think you eat a lot of calories, but until you track it how you will know? Simply put— you won't. The first thing you'll need to do is measure your weight. You have to know what your starting point is. From there, measure the number of calories in everything you eat and record it.

Use Google, My Fitness Pal, nutrition labels, and anything else you can to get an idea of how much you're eating. It'll never be exact, and that's ok. You want to get a rough measurement of how much you're eating. From there, track the calories in the note app on your phone.

This will be tough, but remember your mind, your goals and your strong determination will get you to your long-term goal. Let's go!!

Why Fasting Diet Can Make You Burn More Fat

Just to clarify when we talk about fasting diet what I mean is intermittent fasting where you only fast for 24 hours 2 or 3 times a week. This method is becoming a very popular way to help burn body fat in a short period and to help maintain your weight loss for life.

That said here are 7 ways this type of fasting can help you burn body fat quickly

1. Your Fat Burning Hormones are increased

HGH (Human Growth Hormone) is the most important fat hormone in our body. When we are a fasted state the production of this hormone is increased resulting in higher amounts of fat being

473

burned. Fasting also allows the insulin levels in our body to reduce so you burn fat and not store it

2. You have lots more fat burning enzymes

When you are producing more fat burning hormones then you need a more fat burning enzymes to help them do their job properly. The two most important enzymes that assist in this process are Adipose tissue HSL and Muscle Tissue LPL. Simply explained the HSL enzyme encourages your fat cells to release fat for energy to be used in your muscles and the LPL enzyme has the job of getting your muscles to soak up the fat so it can be burnt for fuel. Fasting increases the release of both these enzymes therefore creating a fantastic fat burning environment.

3. You actually will burn more calories when fasting

I have to admit I was not sure about this claim at first but after a few weeks of my fasting diet I found myself having extra energy and being more alert and awake on my fast days. The reason for this is that short term fasting (12-72hrs) actually boosts your metabolism and adrenaline levels. This combination results in extra calories being used and as we all know the more calories, you burn the faster you can lose weight.

4. Instead of burning sugar you now burn more fat

When you have a meal your body will first burn the carbs then the fat from your food. If you can't burn off this fat in few hours after this food then its going to be stored as fat. When you are fasting there is no other energy source in your body so it has to burn body fat and not the sugar in your blood put there by the food.

5. You can understand what triggers you to eat.

When I made a decision to fast what surprised me most was how aware I became of the triggers and habits that made me eat badly. A lot of my unhealthy eating was down to routine and certain situations and by being able to see these more clearly, I started to break these bad habits. Knowing why and what causes you to eat certain foods is an important step to stopping this reaction can help build better habits.

6. Get control back over what you eat.

By doing short fasts, you do feel better about yourself and get a feeling of accomplishment. If you have issues with food then this positive response can help you build a positive relationship with food again. Being in control of what you eat will make sure you are not as vulnerable to eating all the bad foods that cause to put on weight.

7. You can still enjoy all the foods you like.

Short term fasting allows you to burn fat and ultimately lose weight while still enjoying foods you like. The discipline of fasting means on the other days you can have the foods you enjoy but without the guilt and still lose weight.

With this type of freedom in your diet you are far more likely to stick to the plan because you don't feel restricted. Most people fail to hit their goals because they stop too soon, so being able to be consistent over time is the difference between failure and success.

Dietary and Exercise Considerations for Intermittent Fasting

How will your diet affect your weight loss goals while practicing intermittent fasting?

The weight loss benefit of practicing this kind of cycled eating comes from not only stimulating your metabolism and other bodily processes through fasting but simply from having less time to consume as many calories as you would during a normal day. Most people tend to snack throughout the day, eat at least three large meals, and may even consume calories at night through snacks or drinks. By putting a limit on the length of time that calories are to be taken in, most people will drastically reduce the total number of calories per day. Grazing is a term used to describe the pattern of eating that many women find themselves doing, whether they know it or not. Unrestricted access to food is common in today's culture and is putting you at great risk for over consumption of calories—leading to continued weight gain. If you're someone who is used to this style of constant snacking and unrestricted eating, your body has grown accustomed to being fed all day long. This leads to a continual sensation of hunger and the urge to eat at all times throughout the day, rather than just at meal times. It can take some time to retrain your body and brain to limit hunger signals to the appropriate times of the day. Sticking to your intermittent fasting eating pattern will continue to feel easier each time you complete a fasting cycle.

If you have a normal diet, meaning you eat an average amount of food and don't partake in routinely binge or overeating, you should notice weight loss benefits from intermittent fasting without making changes to the foods you eat. This is one of the greatest perks of following the intermittent fasting "diet"! For many women, a diet has traditionally involved restricting calories for an extended period. Not only is this method of weight loss difficult to stick to—limiting the percentage of those who comply long term—but when you extendedly restrict calories, you create a reliance on high-quality nutrition as well. This is a major hang-up for many people who don't have the time to consistently prepare varied and nutritionally dense meals multiple times per day, as well as for those who are just unfamiliar with nutritional science and nutrient needs. Counting calories doesn't take into account the interactions within the body that are specific to every person and their diet. It can lead to a preoccupation with tracking foods consumed versus calories spent, creating mental stress and anguish—a contributing factor to the stalling of weight loss!

By following an intermittent fasting protocol, you don't have to worry about tracking how many calories you consume and logging your exercise to determine how many you've expended. You don't have to swear off your favorite snack foods, and you don't have to restrict yourself to only consuming nutritionally dense foods that you don't have to prepare or that you just don't like. Following your normal diet but planning it around specific hours will jumpstart your metabolism and ultimately provide the weight loss you've been looking for. Intermittent fasting cycling simplifies dieting and weight loss so that everyone and anyone can lose weight! You don't have to worry about preparing and cooking specialty health foods, purchasing overpriced supplements or meal replacements, or spending hours obsessing over certain foods and denying yourself your favorite snacks and treats.

If you find that during your periods of eating you tend to take in a large amount of junk food or you tend to overcompensate for your periods of fasting, you may want to consider making a few dietary changes to help you lose more weight quickly. While intermittent fasting simplifies dieting by eliminating the need to count calories and follow a strict dieting plan, consuming far too many calories will not provide weight loss. It is a simplified, effective weight loss tool, but it is not a magic solution to eating anything and everything you want in great quantity and lose weight! There is no magic solution, and if a diet program ever promises to be one, you should run the other way as fast as you can! It is a understood concept that too many calories in and not enough calories expended will not lead to weight loss, and depending on the difference between the two can even lead to weight gain. Even with the increase in resting metabolic function from the act of fasting intermittently won't completely negate an abnormally high-calorie diet during the non-fasting hours. When you first begin your intermittent fasting cycle, it may be helpful to keep an eye on the kinds of foods you're consuming during your "normal" days and your non-fasting periods, as well as the quantity. If you feel you may be overeating during these times or choosing mainly high-calorie foods, you can consider making a few dietary changes to fully benefit from the effects of your intermittent fasting cycles.

While not required, you may choose to make changes to your diet to experience the most benefits from intermittent fasting in the shortest amount of time. There are no specific nutritional requirements that the intermittent fasting protocol relies on, but a general focus on foods that are less processed can increase the quality of your calories and result in faster and speedier weight loss.

Weight Training Tips For Faster Weight Loss

You live a fit lifestyle year-round yet sometimes we realize the occasional junk food begins to demonstrate its effects. Being the educated fitness diva, you know it's time to start dieting and cook your workout to achieve your goal.

Be that as it may, for reasons unknown when you decide it's time to lose fat, the first thing we tend to do is bounce onto cardio, and weight training is not prioritized.

Whether this is on the grounds that the calorie-burning advantages aren't recognized, you think weight training is to build muscle and not burn fat, you think you can't focus on lifting and losing fat in the meantime, you don't know how to do an efficient weight training program, or whatever the reason. Some way or another we tend to return the weights on the rack when we want to focus on losing fat.

Although there are many benefits of cardio for fat loss, this article covers the advantages of using various weight training programs to lose fat.

You can never outrun a bad diet with just exercise; therefore, it is necessary to control diet as well in some instances. Exercises themselves have a great effect on your weight loss in the long run. There are two ways how this can go:

•   Exercise more and eat even more, which will result in gaining weight instead of losing it.

•   Exercise moderately and carry on with your diet and you will have an accelerated weight loss.

Muscle Metabolism Boost

First off, you ought to know what you've probably heard ordinarily: "Muscle burns fat." In any case, what does that mean? All things considered, muscle doesn't exactly burn fat, however, all the more precisely muscle raises your Resting Metabolic Rate (RMR).

Adipose tissue (i.e. fat) takes no energy to sit on your body, that is the reason once it's there it will stay there until you exert enough energy to start utilizing it as your energy source. Skeletal muscle tissue is called "active tissue" since it requires energy to maintain itself. To simply sit on your body, every pound of muscle on your body uses around 30-60 calories per day.

Proper Workout and Diet

With the right eating routine and workout, each one is capable of putting on 5 pounds of muscle in a year. If we estimate that your metabolism would utilize 50 calories per day to sustain that muscle, this means you will burn 250 more calories consistently (50 calories/day x 5 pounds). With a pound of fat requiring you to burn 3,500 calories, you will lose 26 pounds in a year without spending an additional moment on cardio. ([250 calories/day x 365 days/yr]/3,500 calories/pound of fat).

Presently as being stressed over fitness, sometimes we brush off this advice since we would prefer not to get "big" or "bulky." Our general public is acquainted with the amount of 5 pounds of fat is. We perceive how our bodies change when we gain or lose 5 pounds of fat. What is unfamiliar to us is the thing that 5 pounds of muscle is. Muscle is substantially more dense than fat.

At most gyms, the trainers have a copy of 5 pounds of fat and 5 pounds of muscle. I encourage you to ask a trainer that works there or the front desk person if you could investigate it. You'll be surprised by the volume difference, and you will see there is no need to worry about adding 5 pounds of muscle.

Post-Cardio Fat Burn

That hour of cardio was great to burn that stored energy, yet when you're done on the cardio machine, you're done burning calories. Weight training, then again, keeps your metabolism at an elevated energy use rate for 60 minutes after you're done. Another bonus to weight training!

Exercise science calls this afterburn effect Excess Post-exercise Oxygen Consumption (EPOC). This means after weight training the body continues to need oxygen at a higher rate.

Weight workout for fat loss

Hit it heavy

Muscle tissue growth is just empowered when pressure is applied to it. If you utilize light weights and do rep after rep, your muscle will never have the stress applied to it that it needs to respond as well. This means although you eat cleaner and are on a reduced-calorie eat less, your muscles won't grow.

Numerous dieters lighten up on their weight since they feel heavy is needed just during a bulking phase, and female dieters particularly would prefer not to lift heavy for fear of getting bigger rather than littler. These are myths no doubt.

Ladies should not shy far from heavier weights because they do not have enough testosterone to get the physique of a bodybuilder.

Lower rep/heavy weight workouts burn more calories during the workout due to greater exertion and will guarantee you won't lose an ounce of precious fat-burning muscle.

This workout uses mostly free weights since machines are designed to target individual muscle groups. This reduces the total amount of muscle required for moving the weight. The exercises will be mostly compound to recruit more muscle fibers to work and discharge muscle building and fat-burning hormones. Likewise, stay on your feet rather than sitting or lying down for whatever number exercises as would be prudent.

Speed it up

Doing higher reps with moderate weight could be beneficial for several reasons with regards to fat loss. The muscle fibers utilized during high reps are slow-twitch muscle fibers. These hold less glycogen; therefore less glycogen will be depleted from the body during the workout. This is critical for keeping the muscles full and the metabolism high.

Additionally, the increased lactate from high-rep training supports growth hormone (GH) output which is likewise a key hormone for losing fat.

Slow-twitch fibers likewise recover faster between sets than quick twitch fibers. This will make it possible for adherence to utilizing shorter rest intervals, and keep the heart rate up throughout the workout; thus burning more amounts of fat.

The same concept of utilizing mostly free weights and compound exercises as the heavy weight workout likewise applies to the lower-weight, high-rep workout above. Therefore, the same exercises can be applied however the weight needs to be adjusted to take into consideration more sets and reps.

Opt for Circuit Training

Circuit training is a half, and half kind of interval training where anaerobic (lifting) is combined with aerobic (cardio) exercise, using higher reps and lighter weights.

In your daily circuit you will do one set on a machine, then move to do a set on another machine, and on like that 'till you finish the circuit, bounce on a cardio machine for 10 minutes, and come back to your first machine, with no rest in between.

Anaerobic and aerobic exercise each provides their own particular unique physiological benefits. A unique advantage that circuit training has is it combines both. Quick twitch muscles are used primarily in anaerobic explosive exercises, while slow-twitch muscles are used primarily in aerobic endurance exercises.

One thing to keep in mind is that you'll use no less than two machines at a time. Keep in mind to be courteous at the gym and just do circuit training during off hours. Gym edict does not permit you to claim more than one station while other individuals are wanting to get through their workout also.

Double Up

Training muscles twice every week benefits from more regular training as well as the split lets you focus on intensity variation. Meaning, the first workout in the week will emphasize heavier weights and fewer reps while the second workout in the week will focus on moderate weight and higher reps.

Go for Supersets

The superset is a super-intensity technique for fat loss and muscle building. With these, you simply do two exercises back to back with no rest in between.

There are several reasons why supersets are more effective than doing the regular one station at a time with rests in between every set.

First, supersets increase Lactic Acid production. Additionally, supersetting is time efficient. By doing sets back to back you reduce your total workout time while as yet doing the same amount of work.

Supersetting involves doing two exercises with no rest in between.

In conclusion, different superset combinations can increase muscle fiber activation. This means you can utilize specific exercise combinations to increase the intensity of work on a specific muscle, helping it develop faster.

Changing Your Mindset

Never aim to lose extra weight by just and making a target of losing certain pounds in your schedules week or month as such approach never works when you are aiming to do exercise on a long-term basis.

Instead, go for exercise to gain more muscle mass and also feel better about yourself overall. As for the fat-losing part, let your diet cover you in the regard.

Don't think of exercising as a formality, do it for your pleasure and to gain confidence in yourself. Focus completely on your diet plan as it is a more important factor in losing weight than hitting the gym. Exercise in such cases is a boost to your weight loss campaign and also a way to keep you away from weakness as a result of weight loss.

Choosing Your Exercise

Lifting and high-intensity intermittent training are the most effective tools for weight loss on the long-term, especially when you are on a meal plan. You will know about both of them in this section.

Weight Lifting or Training

While doing your weight lifting with a trainer, try to focus on your major muscles and never forget about squats. Most of the diets have an effect called 'muscle-sparing effect' which will greatly help you preserve and build lean muscle mass further.

Putting on muscles is not as easy as most of the people think it is, it needs a lot of determination and courage to keep yourself on the same timetable for a long time. Weight lifting will offer you some assistance with building and keep up muscles and burn more calories while resting, as compared to how you did previously. It's a myth that you will develop huge muscles if you lift weights. It takes many years of workout to reach that level.

High-intensity Intermittent Training (HIIT)

This is also called interval running or training. It's a training method in which you interchange intense blasts of anaerobic exercise - for example, sprinting with short recuperation periods. One of the impacts is that you smolder more calories in less time contrasted with other workout schedules, such as delayed cardio.

Don't overdo it

You should exercise regularly, but make sure not to overdo it. Take rest days in between with sufficient sleep to meet your demands. Exercising more than your body is capable will increase the risk of getting injured. Furthermore, it will also negatively affect the immune system and increase hormones that are related to physiological stress, leaving you with more harm than good.

Set Goals

Always set your weight loss goals more than you think you can achieve and for that you will have to work out harder than you did before. You should always aim to lose more than 2 to 3 pounds per week.

If you are using a calorie calculator during your diet plan, do not go for large calorie deficits but try to settle ideally for no more than 500 Kcal and also depending on your basal metabolic rate (BMR) and activity level, shoot for a reasonable energy intake of 1300 to 1700 Kcal.

How to Incorporate Building Muscle During Intermittent Fasting

In recent years, many people have become curious about Intermittent Fasting. There may be a variety of reasons for this increasing interest. These reasons range from wanting to lose fat the easy way, to peoples' busy lifestyles. Many have no inclination to cook multiple meals a day. Some people also have busy schedules where they are unable to squeeze in a lunch or breakfast.

In some cases, Intermittent Fasting is followed by people due to certain beliefs. For example, by Muslims when they fast during Ramadan or otherwise from about 5 am to 7 pm.

Whatever your reasons may be, you may have wondered how you can build up any muscle mass while following this eating schedule. A lot of people assume that it is next to impossible to gain muscle mass while fasting. The fact is that if you spend a little time to plan out your day and your meals in the correct way, you can easily build muscles while fasting!

Here are some of the things that you should keep in mind to maximize your success.

Opt for training sessions that are scheduled late at night

If you are fasting for a specific period where you will be fasting from a set time in the morning to a set time in the evening (for example the Ramadan fasting set up of 5 am to 7 pm), it is best if you place your workout sessions for after 7 pm, as waking up and working out before 5 am will be a Herculean task.

It is always advisable that you consume some food before you start with your resistance-training program, so doing your training session before 7 pm is extremely unlikely. You also need to consume a certain amount of carbohydrates and proteins after your training program is over so that your body can begin the recovery process. You will not be able to do this if you are supposed to be fasting for that particular period.

When you start with a late evening training session, you can make sure that you consume your dinner immediately once you are home from work or as soon as your fasting period ends. This meal can act as a "pre-fuel" before you begin working out.

You can then start your training session, once you are done eating, say at around 7:30 pm and continue training for an hour or however long your workout lasts, giving you time to finish it by say 9 pm. This will give you enough time to squeeze a post workout meal into your schedule until it is time for bed at around 10 pm.

Consume the bulk of your caloric requirement after your training session

The second most important thing for you to do while following this protocol is to be sure that you consume the bulk of your required caloric intake immediately after you finish working out. As mentioned before, this post workout meal helps the body with regeneration. By helping the body to recover from the workout, this post workout meal aids in the generation of lean muscle mass in the body.

For this to work, you first need to figure out the number of calories that you need to consume in a day so that you can build up an adequate amount of muscle mass. Once you figure out your total caloric needs for the day, consume about 20% of the required calories right before you begin working out. This meal should contain both carbohydrates and proteins, as this meal will act as a fuel for your workout. If you do not consume adequate carbs or proteins, you will feel extremely lethargic and tired.

After you finish your daily workout, the post workout meal should consist of about 60% of your total required calories. These calories can also be divided into 2 or 3 small meals in the time span that ranges from post work out to bedtime.

This meal is likely to contain a large number of calories that you need to consume in a short span of time. You may find it difficult to consume the required quantity of calories all together. It helps to focus on consuming foods that have a large number of calories, such as red meat, dried fruit, bagels, raw oats, etc.

You should also keep in mind that the meal you are consuming is immediately after you finish working out. So, with this kind of a meal plan set up, you should consume high carb foods that will help in building muscle, rather than opting for foods that are high fat and low carb. This is because immediately after working out, your body requires carbohydrates. In this scenario, if you provide your body with more fat, it will have a detrimental effect on your body.

This doesn't mean that you have to eliminate all the fat from your diet. You can consume a meal that has a lot of carbs or proteins just after you finish your training and then consume a high fat or high protein meal just before you sleep. The point is to keep the fat consumption low in the meal that immediately follows the workout session.

Fatty foods are more calorie-dense, and it is extremely easy to eat them in a large amount, for example, nuts, butter, oils, etc. These are easier to consume than a lot of high carb foods – especially when you are already feeling satiated. So, it is best if fatty foods are consumed as a second small meal just before bed, while carbs are consumed immediately after working out.

Try to squeeze in a meal before 5 am

The last thing that you need to do while following this approach to building muscle while Intermittent Fasting is to eat a meal immediately after you wake up. For all of the people who aren't following Ramadan and are just fasting to lose weight/gain muscle mass, this meal can be consumed at whatever time you naturally wake up.

If you are following Ramadan, it is advisable that you wake up earlier, say around 4:30 am, just before the fast begins, and consume a slow digesting protein, such as red meat with some cottage cheese, that will make up for the remaining 20% calories that you need to consume.

You can also add in some fat or carbs to this meal, but make sure that you consume about 35% of your required protein at this time. This ensures that there is a steady supply of amino acids in the body while you fast throughout the day.

After consuming the meal, you can go back to sleep if you want.

Make sure that when you follow this type of muscle building Intermittent Fasting regimen, that you keep all of the points above in mind. If you try to perform a large volume of highly intense exercise while consuming very few calories, your body will react negatively to it, and you will do yourself more harm than good.

Slowly, the body will lose all the stored glycogen and will be deprived of it. This will result in lethargy, the inability to keep up with your workouts and the incapability to recover. To be sure that this doesn't happen to you, you will need to force feed yourself until your body becomes acclimated to this meal cycle. Eventually, this approach will start feeling normal to you and your body.

Does Exercise Play a Role in Intermittent Fasting?

As promised, intermittent fasting will produce weight loss for most women regardless of the incorporation of an exercise regimen. Pairing your intermittent fasting cycle with a lifestyle that isn't sedentary will be enough. Not sitting for long periods of time and regular movement are both important factors in any healthy lifestyle and any diet routine aimed at weight loss.

Regular movement and even exercise can be an important aspect of any weight loss plan, but exercise alone won't cancel out continuously poor dietary choices. The foods you consume have a greater impact on the regulation of weight than does your physical activity or fitness.

So, the bottom line is that most women don't need to exercise to lose weight while practicing intermittent fasting, but if you want to incorporate structured exercise into your routine, certain activities can give you the most "bang for your buck." Plus, as an bonus, exercise can be a temporary appetite suppressor, and one study of overweight participants showed that those who engaged in physical activity every other day while following an intermittent fasting program lost more weight than the group that didn't.

The best exercise routine to pair with your intermittent fasting cycle is to visit the gym three times per week and perform a brief warm up, a weightlifting routine, and a few cool down and stretching poses. Now, I know what you're thinking. Don't be intimidated by the mention of exercise or weightlifting. As promised, the addition of regimented physical activity to your cycled eating is optional, and you may find you don't need or wish to incorporate it into your intermittent fasting practices. The beauty of this plan is in its universal effectiveness—it can benefit everyone from body builders to you!

For those who are interested in a workout routine that will optimize their weight loss while following an intermittent fasting eating plan, I've simplified the science behind these specific exercises as well as created an easy-to-follow regimen that will provide you with confidence at the gym. And of course, you don't need to worry about these weightlifting exercises making you appear bulky or muscular; they are specifically geared toward women's bodies and when combined with intermittent fasting, can help you achieve a toned, healthy look!

Lifting weights will burn calories while providing an extra boost to your metabolism (on top of the increased metabolic stimulation intermittent fasting provides.). Studies have shown that even while actively following a diet plan and losing weight, weightlifting can build muscle.

Rules for incorporating simple exercise into your intermittent fasting weight loss routine:

• On the days you are fasting, do a light physical activity like yoga, low-intensity swimming, or light cardio like a brisk walk or slow jog.

• On the days you are not fasting, do a more intense physical activity like high-intensity interval training or weight lifting.

•Drink plenty of water when doing physical activity, on fasting and non-fasting days!

An example of a high-intensity interval training exercise can be as simple as follows:

Three rounds: 20 seconds of exercise and 10 seconds of rest between each exercise.

1.   Air boxing: Stand with your right foot slightly in front of your left and your hips pointed toward your left side. Set your arms in a boxer's stance and

punch with your right arm toward your left side, and then punch with your left arm headed toward your right side. Repeat.

2.   Air boxing (again): Rotate your stance so that your left foot is slightly in front of your right and your hips point toward your right side. Again, take your boxer's stance and punch with your left arm first followed by your right.

3.   Jumping jacks: Simply do as many jumping jacks as you can do in the 20 seconds of allotted time.

4.   Squats: Do as many squats as you can in the 20 seconds of allotted time, ensuring you are squatting deep enough to feel your thigh muscles begin to tire.

An example of a simple weight training routine for women:

A weight lifting routine for women does not have to be complicated, heavy, or produce bulky results. Engaging your muscles in weight lifting activity will keep your bones strong and healthy, lower your risks of osteoarthritis, and build muscle mass, thus increasing the speed of your metabolism and providing you with the toned arms and legs that most women seek. Weight lifting does not always have to include lifting actual weights! Bodyweight exercises are incredibly effective for slightly increasing a woman's muscle mass and shaping her body.

Always warm up before beginning your routine!

Start by doing squats. Try doing somewhere between 8 and 12 squats, take a small rest, and repeat one more time.

Use one light dumbbell in each hand (approximately 8 pounds) to do two sets of rows, somewhere between 8 and 12 rows per set. Stand with your feet apart, in line with your knees, and your knees slightly bent. Keep your back flat and lean forward from your hips. Lift the weights up to your chest while pulling your shoulders back. Your elbows should be bent and pointed backward while your palms face in.

Next, use your body weight to do push-ups. Start out doing them on your knees, and move to a full push-up whenever you feel capable. Again, do two sets of 8 to 12 push-ups, increasing the number as you gain strength and are able.

Finally, end your routine with a plank. To do this, you'll hold your chest off the floor with your forearms, while your toes face the floor. Lower your waist toward the floor until your body becomes a straight line, parallel to the floor. Start by holding this position for as long as you can, eventually working your way up to a 60-second hold.

Don't be intimidated by the incorporation of exercise into your intermittent fasting routine. Increasing your physical activity will benefit your weight loss and provide an even greater boost of energy. Don't feel that you need to start everything at once! You may find it easier to begin your fasting routine for a few weeks before you add in an exercise routine. The most important aspect of any weight loss program is to do what works for you! This will increase the likelihood that you'll stick with it long enough to see results.

What to do about low energy?

Low energy is one of the hardest hurdles to overcome (other than hunger) when you're on an IF diet. The biggest reason for this is that there are many different causes. With hunger, there are defined reasons you could be hungry. Ghrelin and several psychological cues all cause hunger. So what causes low energy? It could be hundreds of different physical factors. So, instead of focusing on what causes hunger, let's jump right into solutions. These solutions include seeing your doctor for bloodwork in case you're low on vital nutrients, exercise, taking a shower, meditation, napping, going outside, and switching your IF method.

Seeing Your Doctor

The first thing that you should do when you're too tired while fasting is to see your doctor. It's very important to rule out a physical cause before moving onto something like exercising. It's not necessary to see a specialist; just your local friendly GP will do. You may want to call ahead of time and check that they've worked with patients on special diets before. Not all doctors will be familiar with the benefits of IF.

After you've found a doctor to see, make an appointment that's most convenient for you. In the time between your appointment and now it may be best to take a break from your fast if you are feeling unwell. Your health should always come first.

On the day of the appointment, your doctor will ask you a lot of questions about your diet. Make sure you come prepared with your medical history, and all of the details of your diet prepared. Your doctor will most likely prescribe some amount of blood work or supplements. They may even suggest some of the things you've already read this book! Your doctor is your partner in your weight loss/health journey, so it's critical that you follow their advice. Be sure to ask your doctor whether or not you can continue your fast while you wait for your test results if he or she has ordered them.

Once the test results are back, your doctor or a nurse may call you back with your results. They may ask you to come back for a follow-up appointment. If your fatigue is explainable by the results of your blood work, your doctor will work with you on a solution suited to your situation.

Exercise

There are many types of exercise out there, but the benefits are all the same - improved health, strength, and the benefit of natural endorphins. Exercise is also proven to provide a natural boost to your energy level. For this reason, IF and exercise usually go hand in hand. However, certain types of heavy exercise that require a lot of energy (calories) should probably be avoided while on a fast. For example, you probably shouldn't run a cross country marathon while also fasting! Here are four great examples of exercise that works well with fasting.

Running

There are hundreds of books, articles, and websites dedicated to the benefits of running. Unless you suffer from a severe medical illness, there are no downsides to running. There are even some anthropologists who argue that the human body was built for long distance running. In fact, some hunting tribes in Africa simply outrun their prey. The prey eventually becomes too tired to escape!

One of the best programs for a beginning runner is called "Couch to 5k". It is free to use and requires no special equipment. You simply run three times a week using a special timed schedule, especially for beginners. The first week's three sessions all start with a 5-minute walk. Then, 60 seconds of jogging. Finally, 90 seconds of rest. Repeat for 20 minutes. That may seem easy to handle, but if you're just starting out, you may be surprised at its difficulty. You can read about the full program on Cool Running's website, coolrunning.com.

The benefits of running to focus and attention were shown in a study by scientists at the University of Illinois in 2003. Twenty men were tested using a device on their heads that measured brain activity. They were measured before and after 30 minutes on the treadmill with mental tests. The areas of the brain known to contribute to focus and attention were significantly more active after the run. You can use these same benefits to your advantage while you fast!

Yoga

Yoga is a mental exercise as much as it is a physical one. It originated in India around the sixth or fifth century BCE. Back then, Yoga was mostly a religious practice. It's come a long way since its origins. Now everyone around the world participates in Yoga for its many benefits. It has a very spiritual core to its practice, but you don't have to believe in anything to try it and experience its benefits. It's been shown to lower risk of heart disease as well as help to energize those who practice it.

The best way to start yoga is to get hands on teaching from a local "yogi" or teacher. They're pretty easy to find through the internet these days - just search "yoga practice [your city here]." You'll get many results!

Another way to start yoga is by doing it yourself at home. You can look up beginner poses online, or even watch videos on popular websites like YouTube that will guide you through everything you need to do. It's best, to begin with small 15 to 20-minute total body yoga sequences before moving onto anything advanced. All you need to begin is a mat. Even a towel will work if you don't have a yoga mat.

It's best to perform your yoga practice at the same time every day. You could even dedicate a certain space in your home or workplace for this purpose.

Swimming

There's nothing quite like jumping into a cold pool of water to wake you up! This, combined with exercise is a great way to wake yourself up if you're feeling fatigued. To top it off, it's cheap! All you need is a local pool and a swimsuit. If you don't already know how to swim, there are many classes offered at local recreation centers. This exercise is best used in the morning or evenings after work. There are many advantages to swimming over another exercise.

Water makes you highly buoyant. When you are submerged up to your neck, you are 90% buoyant. That means that exercise is much easier. You won't hit the floor quite as hard, and you'll have increased flexibility. There's also constant resistance from the water all around you. There's an estimated 12 to 14% more resistance in water than on land. That means you'll be working harder for the same amount of exercise than you would do on land. Lastly, water is great for keeping cool. This makes it a great option if you hate getting sweaty and hot when you exercise.

Besides swimming laps, there are a lot of water exercise options including:

1. Water walking: simply walk in neck deep water.

2. Water aerobics: exercises performed to increase the heart rate for 20 minutes or more.

3. Water strength training: using water exercise equipment, such as floaters, to increase resistance and strength.

4. Flexibility training: increasing your range of motion through stretching.

5. Water Yoga: yoga designed to be performed in a pool of water.

6. Deep water running: simulates running on land with special flotation devices.

Each of these exercises, or even just lap swimming, will increase wakefulness and help fight fatigue.

Dance

Dance is exercise and also my personal favorite! It's particularly good at taking your mind off any stress you might have because you have to coordinate movements and focus. Many exercise classes today even incorporate dance. Ever heard of Zumba? How about Jazzercise? These are two of many types of exercises popular these days that heavily incorporates dance. Dancing is an efficient way to bring your heart rate up, have fun, and get some great cardio in as well. Whether or not you think you can dance well, the movement will be enough to wake you up.

Your first, easiest, and cheapest option is to turn on the tunes and get into the groove simply. You can do this by yourself, or with others if you're confident enough! Since it's only to wake yourself up, there's no reason to worry if you're doing it "right." Brushes make great impromptu microphones if you'd like to sing along.

Your second option is to take a dance class. Simply search online for dance classes near you. There will be many to choose from. These are some of the best types of dance to increase your alertness by raising your heart rate:

1. Zumba

2. Jazzercise

3. Swing dancing

4. Salsa dancing

5. Belly dancing

6. Pole dancing

If you still can't decide on a class, listen to the type of music that would be played in the class. Choose the class for which you like the music best. This will make the class more fun. Therefore you'll be more likely to keep going.

Showering

Showering is something you probably already do in the morning to wake yourself up. If you work from home or have access to a gym with a shower at work, this is a great quick option that you can use on your lunch break. You'll feel cleaner as well as being more alert. If you feel that a full shower would be too much to take, don't worry. You don't need to use soap, shampoo, conditioner, or anything else you normally do in the shower. This is purely for the purpose of waking up. To optimize your experience follow these steps:

1. Step into the shower, and turn on the water to a comfortable temperature.

2. Enjoy the warm water for 5 minutes.

3. After you're comfortable, turn the water to be as cold as you can take it for 30 seconds. The colder, the better. This step is important.

4. After your 30 seconds is up, turn the water to be as hot as you can take it for another 30 seconds. Again, the hotter, the better. This is also important. It will increase your blood flow and stimulate you further.

5. End the shower with one more 30-second bout of cold water. Again, as cold as you can stand it.

This is a form of something called "hot and cold hydrotherapy." It's been around for thousands of years. It reduces stress and increases your tolerance to stress. It strengthens your immune system. The cold water tightens your blood vessels, increasing your blood pressure which is fantastic for your heart's health. And last but not least, it will certainly wake you up!

Meditation

While it's great for focusing your mind on fighting hunger and cravings, it's also fantastic for helping you increase alertness and fight fatigue. This may seem like a bit of a paradox at first. How can something relaxing and calming cause you to feel more alert and awake? You'll be surprised to find out that there have been studies that prove meditation is a great tool for this purpose. More than that, meditation can help you mentally to cope with and become accustomed to your new IF diet.

Stress is a very large reason for why we become tired in the first place. Changing your lifestyle can be very stressful. For that reason, you'll probably be pretty tired when you start your IF diet. The part of your brain that is most active during stressful or tiring events is the amygdala. During mediation, the amygdala decreases its activity significantly. Meditation will help you to manage and maintain this benefit. Often, you may find that your stress was misplaced or based on fear the meditation will help you work through.

Another benefit of meditation is that it has no side effects like sugary energy drinks. Energy drinks, coffee, and supplements are very temporary solutions. And it's dangerous to drink too much in one day. They often leave you feeling more tired than you started afterward. Thankfully, meditation has no side effects! You meditate as much as you'd like with no negatives afterward. In fact, a chemical often used in energy drinks is DHEA. It has been proven that your body naturally produces more DHEA when you meditate. It's a great all natural alternative.

To feel more awake, it's important that you get good sleep. Meditation helps to increase the quality of your sleep. It will make you more mindful in your waking hours so that you go to bed on time and relaxed. This is important for your health in general, but especially while you are fasting and your body is burning its energy resources.

Going Outside

Going outside is a natural and easy option to help with fatigue. Light has been shown to assist with many sleep and mood disorders, such as seasonal depression and delayed sleep phase disorder. Sometimes these conditions are treated with special light equipment. However, all you need to increase wakefulness would be 10 to 20 minutes spent in the outdoors. Going outdoors to do some quick grocery shopping will take your mind off things and can easily add 1-2 hours to your fast.

What Kind of Progress Should You See?

As with any new eating or exercise regime, you can expect there will be some fluctuations throughout your week. While overall you can expect to lose 3-8% body weight (and a bit of your waist!) within your first 3-24 weeks, the important thing to remember is that there may be some up and down to start. However, over time, you should expect to see weight loss throughout your fast, no matter which type you've chosen. The weight loss should be steady, and while some fasts may cause you to lose more weight (because some fasts may cause you to lose muscle, as discussed), you should notice these effects no matter which fast you've chosen.

You should see a decrease in fat and an increase in muscle mass (unless you're doing an extended fast) once your body has normalized. Your clothes will fit differently, you will move differently, and your taste in food may even change as your pallet is cleansed through fasting.

After you've been on a fast for about a week or so, you should notice you aren't feeling as hungry as you used to. Your body has adapted to the new eating schedule, and you should be able to get through your fasts a little easier. In fact, your body will have stopped craving food at times it used to be accustomed to being fed at and now will crave food to the new schedule you have forced it into. This is great progress because it shows your body is adapting and it will then be easier on you to continue your fast.

Your mood will stabilize if you're at the right level of fasting for yourself — if it hasn't stabilized after about ten days, you will need to consider one of the options we discussed earlier: either change your fasting cycle by decreasing your fasting days or decrease your workout intensity.

There's a chance you may have to change what activities you do at what times. Perhaps you aren't focusing as well in the afternoon as you were before. Well, try to move those activities to the morning when you are more critically alert. You should notice increased clarity since you have simplified your eating routine and made the appropriate adjustments to decrease the negative effects of having too much fat on your body (lethargy, trouble focusing, etc.).

How Can You Track Your Progress?

Start by recording your weight before you start your plan, as well as your measurements. Take before photos. This combination is the best way to see your true success from home. If you have a gym membership or access to the coaching staff, you can ask them to help you with these things.

Your doctor can also help you with some important measurements like blood pressure, cholesterol levels, blood sugars, and other specific medical testing that cannot be done at home. If this interests you, then try to book in with your doctor about once a month to keep track of these measurements. These can be some of the better measures of your true health because they are internal factors that are directly influenced by diet and exercise, as opposed to strict body image (just because a person is thin, doesn't mean they're healthy inside; vice versa for someone who is very muscular).

Pick a day and a time that is consistent, week-to-week, to show your true results. As mentioned before, you may notice some fluctuations early on, but this baseline will help you realize the true effects later on. Not only that but if you see a 1-2-pound fluctuation in a week, that is nothing to be concerned about; in fact, that is quite normal.

As your fast goes on, you will now have a baseline and a consistent measurement schedule to help keep you focused and on track. It is important that you eliminate as many variables as possible, so you get the most accurate results possible.

Other, less scientific, ways to measure your progress is to keep track of how you feel each week, both regarding general feelings about the fasting, but also in regards to how you are feeling on a mental and physical level. Notice how your clothes fit differently as the weeks go by. Do you have a particular pair of pants or a shirt that is a little too tight or ill-fitting right now for you to feel comfortable in? Add it to your assessment each week and see how your body is adapting by how that article of clothing is starting to fit. Maybe you are increasing your muscle size, and you have a shirt you need to fill out more — this is the same situation: try it each week to see when it finally looks the way you want to. The pictures help a lot with this because as you go through each week, you can see physical changes you may not notice in the mirror. We look at ourselves a lot during a day, so the captured image of a photo can help us realize the differences when we put them side by side.

Energy levels may also change as you go through the process. They may go up and down as the weeks go on, so keep track of these, too. You may be able to problem solve some issues by reflecting on when you feel tired and how long your bouts of lethargy last. Sometimes caffeine will help you through these times if you find you're truly struggling, or perhaps even a nap. Napping may help get you through some of your cravings and provide you with a mental boost as well.

Weight Loss Effects

Surprisingly, there are positives and negatives associated with losing weight. We have discussed many of the positives already, but some of the negative side effects can be things like loose skin, seeing stretch marks that you didn't notice before, having to buy all-new clothes (this can be an expensive task!), and having to adjust certain medications that depend on hormone and weight balance.

These negative effects can often be offset by patience, determination, and your doctor's assistance.

Once you've figured out that living a healthy, fit life is well-worth these potential setbacks, you will overcome any obstacles set in your path and embrace the new you.

You will likely have more energy and feel more confident than you had before. Your workouts will get more complicated and fun, and you'll notice you're capable of more types of activity than before. With some coaching or personal training assistance, or by doing a ton of research and hopefully getting experienced feedback from someone who knows how to workout properly, you will be able to try new exercises in and out of the gym. This will help you overcome any potential stagnation that can happen when your body adjusts and creates a new homeostasis that you need to work past.

When you lose healthy amounts of weight, you become more trim and fit. You may find yourself open to new experiences like zip lining or scuba diving that you didn't feel confident trying before. Perhaps you'll join that sports team you wanted to but never felt fit enough for. The confidence you will feel by representing your best self, through your hard work and determination will show through when you have adjusted to your transformation. Wear that outfit, try that activity, be competitive with yourself for your personal best in running or lifting.

Preparing for and Preventing Setbacks

Inevitably, you are going to run into obstacles. Some of them are going to throw you off course — sorry, but it is bound to happen! Life is going on around you, and it could throw you a curveball like an unexpected pregnancy (whether yourself or your partner) or a vacation opportunity that prevents you from eating as you had planned. Even if something like this happens, there are some steps you can do to prepare for and prevent some of these setbacks.

Have a backup plan: you may have your heart set on a specific fasting plan, but keep a backup ready just in case. If you are getting off track regularly, the plan you've chosen isn't working for you, instead try your backup plan! Have your reasons ready for why you can't join in a night of drinking, or have that treat. Your friends and family will respect your decisions, and likely appreciate the head's up that you are fasting! You know, just in case you are moody.

Don't put yourself in situations that you know might tempt you until your fast is over. If you know your best friend's birthday is coming up, but you want to do an extended fast, make sure that you have enough time to do your fast and recover from it before that day. Otherwise, have your backup plan ready to go! Try to minimize that kryptonite food you have lying around the house, even now. Are you a chips person? Or maybe a cookie monster? Make it, so you have to consciously plan and act to get these favorite snacks so you are less likely to do so. This will protect your fasting plan and also your waistline.

Plan early and plan often. If you start with a well-rounded plan for your meals and your workouts, you have a better chance of succeeding. Plan them out as far in advance as possible, so you don't have to worry about last minute adjustments — or, worse, so you don't get stuck when you lose your motivation to workout or stick to your fasting regime. Whether this entails planning detailed meals each day for your plan, scheduling your workout and fasting times appropriately, or even creating workout programs for yourself for the duration of your fast, you are in control of every step you take. It may help you to plan all these things, or at least sketch them out so that you don't put yourself in a situation where you have to use your backup plan as your main plan!

Ask for help. Again, tell your family and friends what you are planning to do. If you have a partner, while you shouldn't expect anyone to join you in this endeavor unless he or she wants to, you can ask them to help you through the worst times. Maybe they can do more meal prep, so you don't have to work with food if you're struggling with your fast. Perhaps they can plan your re-feed days with an exciting dinner out together to celebrate your success.

If all else fails, they're a sympathetic ear when the going gets tough.

General Lifestyle Changes

When you decide to add fasting to your way of life, the first thing to remember is that you need a healthy lifestyle. That means including all of the elements included in this chapter. If you do not include them already, then now is the time to start. You will find fasting quite hard if any of these elements are missing from your life, so use these as a springboard because they are necessary.

Exercise

We live in a very sedentary society. That's why a lot of people have weight and mobility problems. In our household, for example, my husband and I were average overweight people whose lives were busy but did not encourage exercise. My husband's mobility problems started years ago, and when we decided to exercise, we took it slowly at first, walking around the yard several times and then increasing that gradually. Don't tell me you can't do it. We were probably the most unfit people you can imagine, and we managed to do it. You have to move the body, or you will find that it's too hard to move out of your chair. Even if you can't do strenuous exercise, start small. Then, we started swimming, and that's a wonderful exercise because it also teaches you to breathe in the right way. There are all kinds of exercises that you can do that are fun and exercise doesn't have to be the dirty word that the public is making it.

If you have a dog, that's a good reason to go for a walk. If you are housebound, you can still exercise because exercise can be done anywhere and these days there are so many apps available that you can even exercise in the privacy of your own home. You need to know that exercise helps you to distribute the food that you eat to the right places in the body and if you simply sit and eat, all of that food will turn into fat.

Water

Drinking water is essential if you are thinking of going into fasting. You should be drinking up to 8 glasses a day, and many people just don't do that. Let's take a look at what water drinking does. Water helps with the transportation of all the nutrients in the food that you eat to all the different areas of the body. It helps to keep your body hydrated, and although you may not put a lot of value on that, let's try and show you what happens when you don't drink sufficient water. Waste and bacteria in the body are not flushed out. There is the risk of illnesses such as colon cancer. Apart from these, the body needs water to keep inflammation at bay, and if you are trying to lose weight by fasting, water is essential. Raw fruit and vegetables also contain water so are helping you to get some water into your system, but if you seriously want to use a detox fasting system, water is vital to the picture. Get used to drinking water and lots of it, but glass by glass, rather than gulping it down in a couple of sessions. You need to have water throughout the day so always carry a bottle with you and if you don't like the taste of it, use flavorings such as a slice of lemon and even make water into green tea for some of the time.

Sleep

You need eight hours sleep a night. If you are unhealthy and want to fast, then you will need all the help you can get from nature. Sleep is nature's way to heal the body and if you deprive yourself of sleep, don't expect to stay on a fast for a long time because you will fail. There are other reasons for wanting to sleep for 8 hours. During the fasting, those eight hours is helping you to pass the fasting period without even thinking about it. That's very valuable indeed if you want to do the fast work for you.

Nutrition

It makes sense that if you were to fast for a period and then eat fifteen bagels, you would still retain the weight that you said you wanted to lose. Be honest with yourself while you are fasting. Fasting isn't a fad. It's a lifestyle choice. You have chosen this lifestyle because you want to lose weight. Although you have a license to enjoy foods, there is a really little point in even trying if you can't be sensible about your food choices. You need to eat a variety of fruits and vegetables and avoid all of those high sugar, high carb foods that you know to be bad for you. Your body needs a certain amount of carbs, but you need to balance out your eating so that you enjoy it but so that it is nutritionally sound as well. I say this because you have to remember that I come from a family of "fatties" and I know all the tricks in the book as far as cheating is concerned. When you cheat, the only person being cheated is yourself.

Conclusion

We have come to the end of the book. Thank you for reading and congratulations for reading until the end.

I hope the book has opened your eyes to the endless ways through which you can lose 3 pounds of fat a week, build muscle, stay lean and feel healthier.

Book 8: Intermittent Fasting

How to Eat what you want and still have rapid weight loss and gain lean muscle for beginners

By

Heather Trill

Introduction

Unless you're one of the lucky few people on the planet who can eat whatever they want but never seem to gain an ounce, you've likely been on a diet or two.

And with so many fad diets to choose from - the grapefruit diet, the cabbage soup diet, the raw food diet and the juice diet, each more bland and painful than the one that came before it – you probably found one that helped you lose a pound or two.

But based on the history of most diets, those pesky extra pounds are likely to be still hanging around, as stubborn as ants at a summer picnic.

That's because most fad dieters find that whilst their latest diet will temporarily help them to drop a few pounds, it doesn't teach them lasting changes, so in al- most all cases, the weight just comes creeping back on again, usually with a vengeful few extra pounds, just to teach us a little lesson.

So, it's back to the books and back to the diets, only to lose – and gain – all over again.

What this book covers:

We will look at some of the benefits that we gain to fasting in addition to what Intermittent Fasting is all about. We will also look at what Intermittent Fasting is all about and what exactly it entails.

If there's one thing experts agree on, that the cycle of yo-yo dieting wreaks havoc on the metabolism, slowing it down to a crawl and making losing weight that much more difficult in the future.

So, is it all over but the crying, and should you just head to the kitchen and whip up a batch of double-fudge brownies and forget about it?

Well, no, don't throw the towel in just yet. There are things you can do to stop the viscous cycle and rev up your metabolic rate again.

With intermittent fasting, you can drop weight quickly, without feeling too deprived along the way.

"For body transformation, intermittent fasting works." This book contains some of the useful tips on how to achieve a successful fast and in the right manner, read on to be enlightened more.

Chapter 1: All about Intermittent Fasting

Intermittent fasting is not a starvation diet. On the other hand, it's also not a way to eat a steady diet of junk food and get away with it. Intermittent fasting is a planned schedule of eating that allows you to eat a normal, healthy diet most of the time, and then requires you to spend a short period of time-consuming far less food. There are some intermittent fasting plans that divide fasting and non-fasting periods into mere hours, such as eight hours of eating followed by twelve or sixteen hours of fasting.

More commonly, intermittent fasts are divided by days of the week.

On the Intermittent Fast Diet, you eat a "normal" diet for five days of the week, interspersed with two days of fasting. Although the research on intermittent fasting is still in the beginning stages, there is sufficient evidence that eating in this way can help to shed fat, regulate some of the hormones associated with obesity and hunger, and even improve overall cholesterol levels.

Because intermittent fasting can have a beneficial effect on the hormones that stimulate fat storage and hunger, it can be a very useful strategy for losing weight and shedding body fat. It can also be a very good way for people who don't otherwise follow a healthy diet to break addictions to foods that are unhealthy and learn to make healthier food choices overall.

On the Intermittent Fast Diet, you eat a healthy diet that is close or equal to your daily caloric requirements for five out of seven days. On the two fasting days, women consume 500 calories per day while men consume 600 calories. Because you'll still be eating during the fasting days, this method of intermittent fasting does not generally lead to overeating on non-fasting days, which can be an unwelcome side effect of other fasting plans.

Fasting isn't something new. Human beings have been fasting for a large part of history due to food scarcity or religious/spiritual reasons. Nowadays people fast a lot less than before, and this is quite logical with all the food we have access to.

Intermittent Fasting, on the other hand, is quite new. It is a new and different way of planning your meals. Research has shown several benefits regarding our health and longevity when you Intermittent Fast. It has shown that it, when done properly, manages our body weight, extends life, regulates blood glucose and a lot more. Normally we are accustomed to eating three meals a day, and maybe even consume snacks in-between those meals. But Intermittent Fasting is different. With Intermittent Fasting you are consciously choosing to skip certain meals. This can be done one day a week, but it can also mean that you skip breakfast every day and that lunch will be your first meal of the day.

There are several ways to do it, but this really depends on your goals.

The meaning of Intermittent Fasting is that you deprive yourself of food on certain points of the day. You will only eat between certain hours, the so-called 'Time Windows'. You will choose these time windows by what suits you best throughout your day. For example, if you choose to eat from 12:00 PM to 08:00 PM, then that will be your time window. You'll make sure that you consume all your calories in those hours and nothing outside of them.

How many meals you eat is also up to you. You can choose to divide all your food between 5 or 6 meals, but you can also choose to eat 1 or 2 meals. Regardless, the main concept is: consuming all your calories between certain hours (your time window). So, Intermittent Fasting is not a diet, it is just a different way of consuming your calories. It has nothing to do with what you eat, but is about when you eat. Of course, you need to eat healthy foods and make sure that you don't overeat in the first place in order to be healthy, but Intermittent Fasting itself provides for great benefits.

Chapter 2: Who to and not to fast

Who Should and Should Not Try Intermit tent Fasting?

Most people can safely follow the Intermittent Fast Diet; however, you should consult your doctor before beginning the diet, since it is not recommended for some people.

People Who Are Not Good Candidates for the Intermittent Fast Diet

In particular, women who are pregnant or nursing should not attempt intermittent fasting. The calorie guidelines for the fasting days are simply too low. However, once you have had your baby and/or have finished nursing, intermittent fasting can help you get your pre-pregnancy body back.

People with type 2 diabetes should not undertake this diet. Although some evidence shows that it may correct imbalances of or insensitivity to insulin, once type 2 diabetes has been diagnosed, fasting is not advised.

People with a history of eating disorders should not go on a fasting diet. If you feel that you may have an eating disorder or that you're at risk of developing one, it is not recommended that you try the Intermittent Fast Diet.

Children and adolescents should not go on the Intermittent Fast Diet. Please consult a pediatrician or nutritionist if you are seeking a weight-loss plan for anyone under eighteen years of age.

People Who Are Well-Suited for the Intermittent Fast Diet

The Intermittent Fast Diet can be a great plan for anyone who is otherwise healthy but would like to lose weight and shed body fat. However, the format of the diet can make it especially beneficial to some specific groups of people.

People who currently eat an unhealthy diet:

People who eat a good deal of fast food, processed foods, and sugar can benefit from the Intermittent Fast Diet's nutritionally balanced approach. The focus of both fasting and non- fasting days is on whole foods: primarily lean meats, fresh fruits and vegetables, low-fat dairy, and whole grains. Many people find that after eating this type of diet for a few weeks, they are better able to appreciate healthier whole foods and have a better understanding of what makes a well-rounded diet.

People who are addicted to sugary foods or empty calories:

Many people become addicted to sugary foods, high-carbohydrate processed snacks, and empty calorie beverages such as sodas and blended coffee drinks, which have lots of calories and little to no nutrition. For some of these people, the Intermittent Fast Diet can have the added benefit of helping them break those addictions. This is not only because of the focus on whole foods but also because of the calorie restrictions on fasting days. When you only have 500 to 600 calories to use in a day, it's hard to justify spending half of it on one cola. After a week or two of living without those foods, many people report that the cravings and withdrawal symptoms sub- side.

People who need an especially simple plan :

Some people just naturally do better when steps and choices are very limited. A diet with too many variations and choices or that requires too much planning and decision- making are often hard for such people to maintain. The Intermittent Fast Diet is simple, straightforward, and mapped out step by step. Because of calorie limitations, the fasting day meal plans are extremely simple, and recipes often have just a few ingredients.

Chapter 3: Myths behind Intermittent Fasting

With all the information regarding fitness and nutrition floating on the web, it can be very easy to lose sight of what is real and what is fiction. The recommendations regarding which diet you should implement varies a lot; many are valid, but there are also some common myths.

Not knowing that those myths are false, people can implement the wrong advice, thus sabotaging their own progress (while having a very good work ethic). Me personally, I get very upset when I see this. I used to be the newbie who would search every forum of the web, getting very excited about implementing the false advice that I would receive. And in the end I would sabotage my own progress.

Eventually I slowly began to see that many myths regarding nutrient and Intermittent Fasting just weren't true. But it was when I found mentors who had the results that I wanted that I fully understood what I needed to do to get the same results as them. To be honest though, to get to the point where I could fully see which advice was false and which wasn't was very time-consuming and frustrating. I want to spare you this process by debunking the common Intermittent Fasting myths. But before I dive into it, let me explain why and how myths are formed:

1. Lack of Knowledge and/or Interest.

With all newly discovered scientific evidence, there are people who want to draw conclusions on it while lacking the knowledge needed to properly do so. In order for them to properly draw conclusions on the results of a particular study, they first need an academic background in that specific field. Most of the time they don't have one, so they simply draw conclusions that are false. Besides that, there are people who have the proper knowledge, but who just repeat the same thing over and over again (while somewhat knowing that it is incorrect).

This usually happens when people lose interest in the specific field they are studying and don't want to put in the effort to properly draw conclusions on a particular result. Another main reason is that scientists are afraid of losing credibility. It is very embarrassing for scientists to admit that they were wrong about a certain subject when they discover that the opposite of what they are preaching is true. Most of the time scientists won't publish their newly discovered results in order to retain their credibility.

2. Social Conditioning

When you repeat a lie enough, it eventually becomes the truth. If you keep hearing something that isn't (or is) true, you will eventually think that it must be true. This is also called social conditioning. Why is that? Because we as human beings don't have enough energy or time to actually test everything out ourselves. We need others to 'invent the wheel' for us, so that we can focus on other, more important things. So, while social conditioning can be very helpful, it can also sabotage us. At some point, when these socially conditioned myths are spread enough, it will be very hard to go against it and discover the truth.

3. (False) Marketing

Supplement, food and fitness companies are constantly trying to sell us products by presenting false information. These companies benefit greatly from people who don't have enough knowledge about fitness or nutrition, because they are easier to manipulate. They use manipulation and lies to falsely promote their products to people who aren't well informed. For example, the grain industry is constantly claiming that you need to begin your day with a healthy (read: filled with sugar) cereal, or the food industry which is constantly saying that you need to feed your body throughout the day benefit from the people who think that they constantly need to buy large quantities of food.

The common myths about Intermittent Fasting are the following:

Myth 1: You Will Be Hungry While Fasting

Most people who hear about Intermittent Fasting for the first time are afraid of being hungry while fasting. While this might be true for the beginning when you try to implement Intermittent Fasting, this will undoubtedly go away very quickly. Why is that? Well, almost everything that we do in our day-to-day lives are formed habits. We have habits so that the body doesn't need to use willpower to do certain things. Having said that, when your body is giving you a signal that you are hungry, it is actually a habit trigger.

Most of the time you aren't really hungry, but because you normally eat at that moment you will receive a habit trigger. When you first implement Intermittent Fasting, it will be difficult to ignore these hunger triggers. This is because it takes around 30-60 days to form a new habit or remove an old one. If you persist for the first 60 days, it will become much easier to ignore these signals and they will even eventually go away. Your body will then send hunger signals to different parts of the day. So, when you start implementing Intermittent Fasting, be sure to ignore the hunger signals you receive outside of your time windows for at least the first 60 days. When you do this effectively, your body will learn to send hunger signals to different parts of the day.

Myth 2: Intermittent Fasting Causes Nutrient Deficiencies

Many people think that you won't receive enough vitamins when you are fasting, but this is not true. When you are fasting, you are 'teaching' your body to eat at certain intervals. By doing this, you will not lose essential vitamins and/or minerals. Besides, the nutrients you lose in a day of fasting are regained again when you eat.

Also, you can take your dose of vitamins by taking pills containing them if you really want to consume our vitamins at certain times of the day.

Myth 3: You Are Starving Yourself On Purpose

Nowadays, we are quick to label 'missing certain meals' as starving yourself. We are accustomed to having food around us 24/7 that we freak out when we skip a meal. Yet I wouldn't call 'skipping a meal' the same as 'starving yourself'.

True starvation is when your body depletes all its fat stores and begins to consume your muscles for energy, which leads to death very quickly.

With Intermittent Fasting though, this is not the case. The fasting periods are very short and you get enough calories from your meals (besides your fat stores) to sustain your energy levels.

Myth 4: Intermittent Fasting Will Have A Negative Effect On Your Weight Training Performance

Another myth brought into the world without real and legitimate evidence to back it up. Research done by several people who were fasting during Ramadan concludes that aerobic activities had an insignificant negative effect on their performance. This is even while being dehydrated, as Ramadan involves restriction of fluids.

More studies that didn't involve the restriction of fluids have found that strength training is unaffected by fasting, even when the individual is fasting for 3 days straight. So, that people think that they can't perform well while in a fasted state is simply not true.

Myth 5: You Need To Eat Small Meals throughout the Day to Keep Your Blood Sugar Levels under Control

Some 'health experts' claim that eating small meals will help you to control your blood sugar. But the thing is, blood sugar levels are well-regulated and maintained when you are healthy. They don't go up and down that much when you go without food for a couple of hours, or even a day.

Also, if you look at it from an evolutionary perspective, it is totally normal to go without food for a couple of hours, days, or even a week. Our ancestors sometimes had to go through times where they didn't have any food available, and this didn't have a big impact on their blood sugar levels. So, the myth that you need to eat small meals throughout the day to keep your blood sugar levels under control is simply not true.

Myth 6: You Will Mostly Lose Muscle and Little Fat When You Fast

The exact opposite is true. Fat is a high energy molecule and it contains far more energy than protein (it is around 2 times more energy dense than protein). Therefore, it makes sense for the body to first use the stored fats as an energy source than protein. Also, the primary purpose of fat is to be an energy reservoir for us when food is scarce.

The proteins in our muscles contain a lot less energy, so it isn't efficient for the body to use protein as an energy source. Also, the main purpose of protein is more critical for our skeletal muscle and for our bodies to function properly instead of providing the body with energy. Additionally, if you compare the calorie reserves that are in fats and proteins, you see a tremendous difference. About 85% of our calorie reserves are in fat stores and 14% of protein. Obviously, fat is the most important energy storage molecule. So, from a physiological standpoint, it makes sense for our bodies to first go to our fat stores for energy when food is scarce.

Myth 7: It Is Bad For You When You Skip Breakfast, And It Also Will Make You Fat

It is true that people who skip breakfast are more likely to be fat. This is due the fact that most breakfast skippers have inconsistent eating habits and show a lot less concern for their health. Another reason why people who skip breakfast are heavier than those who don't, is that people who skip breakfast are more likely to be on a diet. And being on a diet can lead to binge eating. Also, people who diet tend to be heavier than non-dieters in the first place.

Therefore, it is logical that most people think that skipping breakfast itself makes you fat. But as explained earlier, it is what breakfast skippers do besides skipping breakfast that makes them fat, and not the actual skipping of the breakfast itself.

Myth 8: Fasting is bad for women

Some people like to argue that Intermittent Fasting is bad for women. People think that it can negatively affect hormone levels and glucose tolerance as well as lead to decreased satisfaction and frequent hunger in women. While some studies support that theory, other studies have shown that women may continue practicing Intermittent Fasting without any effect on their bodies or hunger levels.

As a woman, I can attest that sometimes, I am just sick of dieting, but that has something to do more with when I was counting macronutrients and my calorie intake than my practicing Intermittent Fasting. I love Intermittent Fasting. I have more control of how much I take into my body and feel like I am able to achieve more satisfaction with my meals if I can intake more due to my fasting throughout the day.

Do I miss eating breakfast? Not really. I miss eating breakfast foods at fast food restaurants, which are bad for you anyway. I can still eat breakfast foods for dinner or lunch if I want. Sure, I cannot get that chorizo biscuit from Carl's Jr that may be bad for my body and daily calorie intake, but I can always make something like it at home for cheaper with fewer calories. I prefer skipping breakfast anyway so that I can train fasted and not worry about packing or making breakfast before work. Who needs extra work in the morning? That is just time taken away from me playing with my phone or sleeping in!

Myth 9: Fasted Training is bad for you

There was a time when people thought fasted training was great for burning fat, especially if you -

are performing cardio. Professional weightlifters were worried that fasted training can cause catabolism, which is the breaking down of muscle. This is also the reason why some athletes attempt to consume something about 30 minutes after a workout so that they can meet a "metabolic window."

Recent studies have showed that even 60 minutes of running while fasted will insignificantly affect your muscle growth. Fasted training will not negatively affect your strength performance as once was thought. However, there is still some unease when it comes to fasted weight training due to the ability to synthesize protein. To help aid in the synthesizing of proteins, it is recommended to consume up to 10mg of BCAA (branched chain amino acids) before and after weight training.

Myth 10: Eating Large Meals at Night Will Make You Gain Weight

You may have heard this saying before: "Eat like a king in the morning, eat like a prince for lunch, and eat like a pauper for dinner." What does that even mean? It basically means eat your smallest meals at night and your biggest meals in the morning. The idea is that consuming large meals at night make you gain a lot of weight. While, eating large amounts of carbs at night will make you weigh more in the morning than if you were to consume just protein; that is only due to the fact that consuming more carbs means your body will retain more water.

More carbs mean more water weight. That makes sense, doesn't it? Carbohydrates tend to hold onto more water than proteins or fats. Recent studies have shown that consuming large meals at night does not make you gain more fat. Actually, recent studies have shown that your meal times do not matter. Have you not eaten throughout the day? Then feel free to eat at night. If you feel like just fasting throughout the day and eating one meal at night, feel free to. The professional competitive eater, Sonya Thomas, also known as The Black Widow, consumes one large meal at the end of a day instead of small meals throughout the day. You may think that competitive eaters are heavy set individuals, but she will definitely surprise you.

Chapter 4: Benefits of Intermittent Fasting

As they were some benefits of the fasting, there are people who are utilizing this to lose excess weight plus some are using it to raise their health problems. Some individuals also say that fasting is a strategy to look young and possess a longer life. This is why that this procedure sounds intriguing to my opinion. The simple fact is that same reasons why I would like to reveal the intermittent fasting benefits together with you.

Really, this ingesting style isn't that challenging. Accusation in court is essentially eating whatever you need within a day and then the overnight you are likely to fast. It indicates no food! (Besides water).It is very completely different from our usual eating habits. However, you can see it as being an extreme weight-loss but fasting is really a great means for anyone to search and feel great inside and outside!

Periodic fasting can help clear up the mind and strengthen the body and the spirit. Although people commonly believe that depriving yourself of food for too long is unhealthy for you, scientists have proven that Intermittent Fasting provides many benefits.

1: It Removes Food/ Sugar Cravings

A lot of the time when we feel "hungry" we actual feel cravings for sugars and carbohydrates. When you are fasting, your body will switch from using carbohydrates as fuel to using your burned fat stores instead. Your body will learn that carbohydrates aren't needed for energy and that it can use the fat already stored in your body for energy.

Aside from removing your sugar cravings, you will also remove the cravings for the food itself.

Because your body "will realize" that it doesn't need food for energy, it won't crave it too often. Thus, by removing all the hunger triggers you'll get through the day. This is why the myth of "eating 5-6 times a day" is not true. When you eat 5-6 times a day and even implement carbohydrates, you'll never allow your body to burn fat. This is due the fact that the body will use the carbohydrates as energy first before using the fat in your body.

2: It Raises Insulin Sensitivity

Insulin is a hormone in the body that regulates the function of cells. Insulin is made by the pancreas and is secreted when we eat food. It then binds to signal cells and allows our body to store the sugars as energy. The less insulin we need to store these sugars, the more sensitive we become to insulin, and the better insulin can do its work in the long term.

When we eat 5 to 6 times a day, our insulin levels stay too high for a long period of time. This insulin won't be used effectively, and this will eventually raise our resistance to it. When we are resistant to insulin, we can develop type 2 diabetes or prediabetes. Diabetes is a disease that prevents us from storing all the sugars we consume, because the insulin that our pancreas produces won't work properly. When this happens the sugars will not be stored as energy and will remain in our bloodstream, leading to high blood sugar levels and hardening of the blood vessels.

This can eventually cause kidney diseases, heart attacks, erectile dysfunction, and loss of vision, strokes, nerve damage and much more critical health problems. However, when you fast for a long period of time, you are forcing your body to use the fat stored as energy and not the food that you are digesting. This will allow your body to create less insulin and therefore become more insulin sensitive, preventing all these problems.

3: It Is Very Simple Intermittent Fasting is very simple.

It doesn't require much effort to plan the quantity, quality and timing of your meals. Any active gym practitioners put much effort in preparing their meals to track their calories. This method is fine by itself, but can be very energy draining and time consuming.

In this day and age, we don't have much time anymore due to our fast-paced, demanding lifestyles, so it is better to save time by eliminating unnecessary duties like meal prepping. When you are fasting you only need to worry about 1 or 2 meals, and you always know at which times of the day you are going to eat. This will allow you to spend a greater amount of time on more important tasks.

When you realize that meal prepping is not so important, you will notice that you are still getting the same results with less effort. This is also called the 80/20 principle. 80% of our results come from 20%

of our efforts. It is up to us to find out which 20% matters. And often, meal prepping doesn't belong to the 20%.

Also, because you are eating one or two large meals a say, it won't be necessary to constantly keep track of your calories. And it is much more difficult to over consume your daily calories in one or two meals (unless you are eating junk food of course).

Note: If you are a professional bodybuilder, then this doesn't apply to you. You can't expect to enter competitions and win them while not staying as lean as possible. So, for those people who are entering competitions, I highly recommend that you keep track of all your calories and stick to what works!

4: It is Flexible

Having strict meal plans can be very difficult to sustain. Most of us have important and demanding jobs that don't allow us to eat when we need to. Rather, we get breaks at the moments that we don't really need them. Or we are traveling a lot, which keeps us from eating our meals when we need to. Fasting, however, provides a huge amount of flexibility. Because you have a short time window, you can choose when to eat. This will give you the opportunity to eat when it suits you best.

For me personally, it becomes really hard to plan my meals and stay on track of my meal schedule when I am traveling or working. Fasting allows me to go without eating for a long time and simply eat when it suits me best.

5: Health Benefits

Studies show that Intermittent Fasting has many health benefits. Individuals who are overweight or suffer from diseases like diabetes may benefit the most from Intermittent Fasting.

Overweight people or individuals with type 2 diabetes will lose more weight and improve their heart health when they fast occasionally. Even if they don't reduce calorie in- take (but rather stay in maintenance mode), they will see results. But of course, if you want to maximize your results, make sure you're in a small calorie deficit and eat healthy foods.

Other health benefits are:

- Limiting inflammation

- Reducing blood pressure

- Improve pancreatic function

- Protects against cardiovascular disease

- Reduce total cholesterol and LDL levels

- Improves insulin sensitivity

While Intermittent Fasting itself is healthy for diabetic people, it can be harmful due to the fact that you are depriving yourself of nutrients at certain times of the day. So again, Intermittent Fasting is healthy for you if you are diabetic, but be sure to consult your doctor first!

6: Rapid Weight Loss

As stated earlier, normally you'll receive energy from the carbohydrates that you consume. This will prevent you from burning the fat you have stored in your body. Yet when you are fasting, you are forcing your body to use the fat you have stored for energy. This by itself will lead to instant and rapid fat loss, which means that you will not only look better, but actually be healthier too.

Also, because you are fasting for 1 or 2 days every week, you are automatically cutting many calories (1000-4500 calories a week). This will result in massive and rapid weight loss, allowing you to lose approximately 0.5-1 pound a week! You will be able to keep your muscle and lose the fat, resulting in amazing body transformations.

7: Improves Brain Health

Intermittent Fasting also has many benefits for the brain. It improves your memory functioning and accelerates learning. It also boosts your BDNF (Brain Derived Neurotropic Factor), which in turn builds your brain tissues. This will make you smarter and help you gain stronger muscles.

Some other benefits are:

Prevents Depression

Researchers have shown that having low BDNF is linked to depression. Good against Alzheimer's Disease Research was conducted with 2 mice with Alzheimer's disease. One was Intermittent

Fasting and the other mouse followed the standard diet (both were consuming the same amount of calories).

They were put in a Morris water maze, and the mouse who was Intermittent Fasting found his way much faster than the other.

Increases Ketone Production

Intermittent Fasting actively stimulates the production of ketones. Ketones are acids that are made by the body to help it use fat as an energy source instead of using carbohydrates as an energy source.

Effective against Brain Trauma

Fasting reduces the mitochondrial dysfunction, oxidative stress and cognitive decline that usually result from brain traumas.

Prevents Huntington's Disease

This disease will deplete your BDNF levels, but research showed that fasting rats with Huntington's disease kept their BDNF levels stable.

Detoxification

It is intended to cleanse the human system of toxins that accumulated during rapid fast-food and heavy meals.

Chapter 5: Does Intermittent Fasting really work?

Intermittent fasting is intended on allowing your body to be hungry enough to consume from stored energy without being in starvation. Starvation mode is when your body has lacked calories for so long that when you do eat instead of using the energy the body will immediately store it in reserves just in case another starvation happens. This is why the fad of "yo-yo dieting" was so unsuccessful – people put themselves into starvation and would actually gain weight once they began eating again. This is also why it is important to have a proper fasting schedule since you want to avoid starvation mode.

Research into weight loss has been around since the 1920's. Studies involving fasting have shown the same results with everything from fruit flies to monkeys. Fasting actually affects what you lose. Most diets will cause you to lose fat, water and even a little muscle but intermittent fasting has been shown to actually concentrate your weight loss on fat alone. It does this by choosing where the best energy source is during your fasted state. Normally your body would choose glucose in the bloodstream or temporarily stored glycogen in the liver since they are easier to process.

When you fast these become unavailable which forces the body to choose the only other stored energy available – fat. This is especially true with working out. If you have tried to drink protein shakes before a workout and have not noticed any improvement this is because your body is choosing to consume the shake rather than any excess body fat you have. Working out in a fasted state forces the body to consume fat to keep up your energy levels.

When you fast, in addition to making your body burn fat you also increase your sensitivity to insulin. When we think of insulin most people think of it as something diabetics need, the reason they need it is because either their body has become desensitized to their own or they are not producing enough. Insulin regulates the amount of glucose in the blood and those who are overweight often find their levels are not right because the body produces so much that it becomes desensitized. By fasting we can increase the sensitivity since your body is being deprived of the readily available glucose it would have from eating too often.

This is a very important tool since with desensitization your body may choose to store more of the glycogen it's making rather than burning it causing your blood glucose level to fluctuate in ways it shouldn't. As the problem of obesity grows worldwide the amount of research into dietary phenomenon grows also. Fasting has its own plethora of science behind why it really does work. So what happens on a day where you don't fast?

The regular intake of food allows the body to keep using the glucose in the bloodstream as it is energy source. Insulin sensitivity will be at normal (or in some cases desensitized) levels. Easily processable glycogen stores will be full which means any additional energy the body receives will go into storage as fat. It won't matter if you eat 20 calories or 200 over your needed amount, anything excess becomes fat and your body has no need to consume any stored energy.

Fasting can be seen as a training method, you are training your body to be more efficient in how it consumes the nutrition you give it. The physiological reasons alone are good enough, but what about the benefits that also come from losing weight? Those who weigh less enjoy a much lower risk for a variety of different health issues, they're also seen as socially superior (something controversial but unfortunately true) and the emotional benefits of having lost excess weight can also lead to an overall happier life. Weight loss can also lead to improvement in other areas – heavier people find they have bad knees or back issues from the strain of carrying extra weight.

The advantages of fasting which might be stated earlier are just the typical ones. The fact in this is a part of the benefits that are mentioned above is always that each individual who have advantages from fasting a result of the belief that everyone is exclusive. And absolutely, each individual who will about to fast will get the matter that he/she desires to be!

Intermittent fasting has grown to be quite the sensation right now. You can find were recent reports that showed that with somebody that has tried it, they dropped a few pounds, and increased how much their own health. Simply to present you with a perception, intermittent fasting is a style of eating where you stand likely to alternative your intervals of fasting, oftentimes only having water as well as on the opposite hand, non-fasting is simply eating precisely what you choose no matter how fatty food is.

Quite simply, a person can eat all sorts of things he wants throughout a 24-hour period and fast for the following 24 hours. This technique to weight control is based on the research along with the ethical practices across the world. When the person will going to present an intermittent fasting he then will certainly get what he could be wanting.

You are likely to notice that there are numerous kinds of intermittent fasts. You can find that we now have 2 kinds of intermittent fasting these are the commonly used as well as the easiest. First could be the daily fasting in which the person only grows to take in once just about every 20-28 hours within a 4-hour period. The second reason is fasting for 1-3x every week, also referred to as different day fasting, when a man or woman eats anything he desires on a single day along with fast the entire of the following day.

Intermittent fasting has many beneficial effects as tried on wildlife like animals and also primates. A report finds out that a man who does the fasting will about to decrease the levels of insulin that he's having and will about to improve the resistance of the neurons inside the brain. In 2008, a survey was developed about intermittent fasting plus it established that the lifespan of an individual improves of 40.4% and 56.6% in C. The public that does the various day fasting has indicated that they tend to give up more weight as opposed to ones who are getting the normal diet. Along with the 2009 study showed that intermittent fasting around the rats improved the rats' survival after having a continual heart failure via pro-angiogenic and then these people have a lengthy lifespan also.

The study only caution is usually that there are few studies which have been completed to the people who do intermittent fasts. The results with the upper frequency within the composition of the body and workouts are interesting and not yet explored in your community of research. However, there are many positive results. Very last month, a study that had been made by the National Academy of Sciences posted a book that ensures that reducing calories 30% per day will planning to increase the memory perform from the old people. In the past year 2007, the journal Free Radical Biology & Medicine indicates to the public the fact that those who are having to deal with bronchial asthma who quicker had much fewer symptoms and in addition they reduction in the markers in the blood that they're having in comparison to the first.

Chapter 6: Nutrition and Training

A major part of Intermittent Fasting is eating. Yes, that sounds self-explanatory, doesn't it? Let me explain. Eating is very important in our day-to-day lives and we must consider what we consume very carefully. With Intermittent Fasting, you can consume higher calorie foods like that six-dollar burger from Carl's Jr or that pasta from Olive Garden without worrying too much about excessive fat gain, but you do have to ensure that your body gets its proper nutrients.

Even though you are using Intermittent Fasting for some flexible dieting, lower calorie foods with a high nutrition profile will help you feel full longer. It is that fiber that fills your stomach! And well, fiber also gets your system moving, if you know what I mean. If you are practicing the Alternate Day Diet or the 5:2 diet, you will find that if you consume a burger for your 500 calories, you will starve before you sleep. Yeah, that burger may taste great, but it will not fill your stomach enough. Plus, you will not get to eat the fries!

How can you get a burger without fries? On the days when you need to consume about 500 calories, it is best to consume 500 calories in vegetables because you will fill your stomach up and feel satisfied. I do not know about you, but most of the time, if I eat a small meal before bed, I will not be able to sleep. I need to eat to sleep! It sounds funny but it is true! As I mentioned in the previous section, you can still lose weight when you consume "bad" foods, but what is important is that you eat fewer calories than your body burns in a day. Do not let food consume your thoughts. If you want to eat out, go for it, but also make note that you should make healthy choices or eat healthy foods the rest of the day.

Eating junk food all day may sound appealing but the sugar and salt will definitely have you buzzing more than if you had been drinking.

Speaking of drinking, try to avoid drinking your calories. Those go by fast and you will miss them when they are! Sure, you can have a Starbucks Frappuccino, but have you seen how many calories are in one? Or how much sugar is in it? My favorite drink, the caramel ribbon crunch Frappuccino, in a Venti size without whipped cream can be over 60 grams of sugar. Seriously, beware!

Also, it is really important to remember that while alcohol can be great, it can have some negative side effects. Alcohol is an empty calorie drink which means it does not help your body run at all. You are just drinking calories! It does not even become usable energy for your body to use! Another important note to keep in mind is that alcohol does eat muscle. What does that mean exactly? If you drink alcohol, it can eat away at your muscle and make you actually lose muscle. Is that not sad? You put all that work into gaining some sort of muscle mass, do not ruin it by downing your body weight in alcohol, all right? That is just not a smart move, especially since alcohol does have calories. They do not just burn away as empty calories!

Here is a special tip: If you are going to work out in the morning or while fasted, consume a cup of coffee or caffeine. A cup of coffee before any exercise routine will increase your metabolism and cause you to burn more when you workout.

Plus, it gives you that energy boost you need to keep working hard. Is that not a great tip? My favorite drink from Starbucks is from the secret menu called "The Black Widow" (not to be confused with the competitive eater) which is just iced black tea and iced black coffee. It will give you a great kick and suppress any appetite you might have until you finish fasting. You are welcome! People who are devoted to their physical fitness or people who want to lose weight may want to include physical fitness training into their daily schedules.

One aspect of physical fitness training involves weight training, which is essential for building a faster metabolism because while the body is at rest, it will burn more if the body contains more muscle. That means you are able to eat more to maintain your body weight! Who does not want that? If you lift weights that are heavy enough to create some difficulty for you, you can build more muscle and even get your heart pumping. An elevated heart rate means you are burning more!

Here is a little advice for you, just because I care: Do not forget leg day! First of all, the muscles in your legs are amongst the largest in your body. You know that muscle you loved to say as a child? Yes, the gluteus Maximus! The gluteus Maximus is the largest muscle in the body. If you do not work it out, you are missing out on training one of the major muscles and you are severely limiting your metabolic potential!

Do not handicap yourself by forgetting such a great muscle. Second of all, have you ever seen those guys at the gym that workout their upper body almost every single day but look a little off kilter? Yeah, well, they forgot leg day. They typically have skinny looking legs that make their bodies so off balance. I have a friend who only works out the muscles he sees so typically his legs and certain parts of his upper body are smaller.

Do not be that guy. Do not forget to evenly train your muscles! Balance is key! It gets a whole lot harder to fix that once you have developed a lot in one area but are underdeveloped in another. Performing cardio is also essential to weight loss. It can create a large calorie deficit if you put the effort into it, but it is also very good for your heart. Heart health can be maintained by proper cardio. While I do not agree that you should utilize cardio for your weight loss because a number of dislike people have associated with cardio which will only lead to more distaste for cardio in the future, I do believe that cardiovascular fitness in maintaining proper health so even if your goal is not to lose weight, I think it is important to continue performing cardio, but in moderate quantities.

Do not make yourself hate cardio by forcing yourself through long episodes of cardio workouts, which I know all too well. Studies have gone back and forth on many aspects of physical fitness and weight loss, but if you want to optimize your fat loss, perform your cardio after your weight training. If you perform your weight training after your cardio workouts, you may find you have expended most of your energy so you cannot properly perform as well as you could have. Although it is important to warm up your muscles, do not tire them out with a long cardio workout.

Aside from optimizing your workouts, if you do perform your cardio workouts after your weight lifting workouts, your body has been proven to burn more fat than if you were to reverse the order of your workout, so if the idea did not entice you at first, at least you can look forward to burning more fat with this workout routine!

Think of that as a secret workout life hack! You are welcome! Of course, your body does require a certain amount of calories to properly operate. If you are at a constant caloric deficit while weight training, all you can attempt to do is keep the amount of muscle you have. You will not be gaining any muscle through a caloric deficit, so if you are trying to lose weight, you will find at the end of your weight loss period, your body will gain weight on the same amount of calories you were consuming before when you were maintaining your weight.

It is a very sad fact of dieting. An important note to take is that you should not be training extraneously when fasted. That is not to say that you cannot work out when you are fasting. Studies have gone back and forth regarding fat loss with fasted workouts. Like I said earlier, all that matters is if the calories you expend is more than the calories you intake. If your body does not perform well starved, do not work out fasted! It works for some but not all. If you do train fasted, though, you should make sure to eat a proper meal sometime after you train.

Make sure that your meal is balanced so you have protein or muscle repair and carbohydrates for energy. While I do not truly believe that your muscles can become "catabolic," it is important to eat to restore your energy. I hate when I feel completely fatigued the rest of the day after working out! I did state earlier that I do train early mornings before work, but still continue to fast after. I have not noticed a large amount of muscle loss at all unless my intake decreases drastically. I prefer to work out in the mornings because the gym is less crowded, I can just get my workout out of the way and go on with my life. Also, statistics show that if you schedule your workouts in the morning, you will most likely perform them compared to if your workouts are in the evenings, which, through experience, I can attest to.

Anyway, I fast until later in the day to prevent myself from binge eating. Training fasted also makes my cardio sessions easier since there is nothing to hinder me or make me feel lethargic. This was mainly through trial and error, but that is how my body responds. Like I have expressed often throughout this book, you should do what works best for your body! All of our bodies do not function or react the same! With that in mind, you must tailor your workouts according to how your body reacts. Some people develop certain body parts a lot faster. For me, my calves develop fairly quickly, which I can tell by the immense pain in my shins when I run. Some people's glutes may grow faster, but some people may not grow muscle easily at all.

This does not just apply to muscles. Some bodies just burn fat faster and not gain any easily, while others gain fat quickly and cannot even get the fat off. It just is not fair, is it? You just need to figure out what type of body you have and figure out what types of workouts work best for you. We may not be all gifted genetically, but that does not mean we cannot do anything about it!

Chapter 7: Intermittent Fasting Types

Intermittent fasting can take several forms. The person designing the method usually determines the difference. However, the factor of fasting and eating will be the constant. All methods have their rewards, so it doesn't really matter, which method you adopt. Therefore, go for the one that you feel more comfortable with and that you feel you can achieve.

The probability of you adhering to the rules is higher if you pick one that you are comfortable with. For beginners, it is advised that you go for a shorter fasting window and a longer eating window. Your body might take between two to four weeks to fully adapt to the new eating system and this is the point where you have to be strong to resist temptations and avoid all those cravings.

Most individuals are already used to eating whenever it suits them so engaging in IF can be really stressful especially at the starting period. Your appetite will naturally lessen once your body adapts to the new eating system. You will also feel a lot slimmer, energetic and alert as you go further. Here are some of the IF techniques:

Fasting Method Number 1

Martin Berkhan designed the first one. His method is quite easy to maintain and very popular. The rule of his technique is that women and men will have 10 and 8 hours eating window respectively, thus leaving them with 14 and 16 hours fasting window. Positive results can be hindered by inconsistent feeding windows thus it is vital to maintaining the windows.

Martin is of the opinion that meals should be consumed around the workout periods. For instance, if 7 pm is supposed to be the end of your feeding window, 5:30 pm should be a good time for workout and meals. Or you could end your fasting windows with workouts that way, you will be able to consume the nutrients required to replenish lost ones just after your workout.

Fasting Method Number 2

The next technique is the Ori Hofmekeler's Warrior Diet. This method could be considered more difficult. In this technique, you are only allowed to eat once a day, which is at night. You are expected to fast for 20 hours per day. Presumably, our ancestors survived doing this.

Although it is impossible to know for sure whether our ancestors did this or not, this method remains very effective. Major positive differences have been recorded by individuals who have engaged themselves in this method. This method might not be the best to start off with; however, the Marin's method would be better for beginners and after a

609

while, you can reduce your eating window till you have just 4 hours left.

You must understand that this method does not allow for small in between meals and as such, don't dive into the deep end of the pool only to struggle to keep up with the 4 hours of eating window. There are certain guiding rules on what you can and cannot eat. This is one of the stricter methods of Intermittent Fasting and as such, you will have to maintain the approved food options, this method is very difficult and as such it is not recommended as much as the others.

Fasting Method Number 3

The third is the method designed by Brad Pilo and is known as the Eat Stop Eat method. This program is a bestseller on the internet. This method basically asks that a complete 24 hour fast be done 2 or 3 times in one week. During the period when you are not fasting, you are allowed to eat whatever you wish. Doing this, you will consume fewer calories and lose weight as a result of this. You can still eat your favorite foods; however, it should be on a day that you are not fasting.

For those who do not want to let go of their favorite meals, this is a huge relief. Notwithstanding, it can be really difficult to go for 24 hours without food. Just as stated earlier, Martin's method is very good for beginners from where you can work your way up.

How do you decide among these methods?

The fact that a method works for someone around you doesn't mean it will work for you. Tailor your fast to suit yourself and while doing this, you must take into consideration your job requirements, sleeping patterns, eating habits etc.

It is always better to allow your sleeping hours fall within your fasting window and you can wait up to six hours after waking up to start your eating window. That is if you are into Martin's method. Some other social commitments can make IF really difficult to maintain.

Whether you like it or not, your social life will be affected by your fasting. Here, you need to be smart to make it work for you. Take for example, Hugh Jackman was on IF while practicing for the movie – Wolverine. Despite the rigors of such schedule, he stuck to his IF program.

It often feels like torture and some people give up and just grab something to eat. This can lead to a feeling of guilt or it may leave you feeling like you failed. They have failed because their goals were not realistic. Setting reasonable goals and marking measurable success is vital to achieving success.

Chapter 8: Intermittent Fasting Plan

The fact that various people have different needs makes it extremely difficult to give you an IF plan. However, you can use the following guides to plan your program.

Know Your Goals.

You should be aware of your calorie number and how many calories you are to consume in order to maintain the caloric deficit of about 500 per day, that is if you want to adopt the IF plan. You are to maintain a caloric surplus if you wish to build your body; however, all calories needed must be consumed during the eating window. It is harder to consume lots of calories because of the time frame by which you have to consume the food but if you are able to consume a lot of calories it is not likely that you will gain fat, if you are in the intermittent fasting program.

You can continue eating what you are eating at the moment if you are okay with your weight level, just ensure your meals are consumed during the eating window. In other words if you want to maintain your current weight but get healthier, keep the same calorie intake that you currently have but adopt the intermittent schedule. If you want to lose weight adopt the intermittent fasting program and reduce your current calorie input by 500 calories. And if you want to gain muscle, make sure that while exercising you maintain the intermittent fasting program and increase your calorie intake by 500 calories a day.

Know Your Schedule.

Timing is the major focus of intermittent fasting and not particularly what you eat. For you to effectively do the IF plan, your eating period and cut-off time must be strictly adhered to. The eating and fasting windows usually control the lives of those involved in IF. They constantly have to check their time and plan accordingly.

Proper planning can help to avoid all these inconveniences. Consider your preferences and schedule: When do you get out of bed? When is the lunch break at your office? Would you rather fast before night sleep or after the morning after the night sleep? You can design your eating window to start 6 hours after you wake up if you would rather go to bed with a full stomach. What happens when you get hungry at work? Will you have the opportunity to take a break and have a meal when the eating window begins? You must consider all these before setting your IF plan.

How Many Meals Will You Eat?

Whatever you like, factor it into your plan. Some would rather have one or two big meals during their eating window while some others may prefer to eat little meals all through the eating window. When Are You Working Out?

A regular exercise program is advised. However, you must factor this into your plan. Do you want to train on a full stomach or on an empty one? It is usually better to have your meal after workouts because this way, the body can regain lost energy and the fuel needed for metabolism can be obtained from the meals.

Chapter 9: Methods of Intermittent Fasting

It is generally accepted that there are 5 methods that can be used for effective fasting. These have either been put together by diet gurus or by scientists and are thought to be effective for their own reasons. As everybody is different it may be that you find one method more appealing than another or that one method will work better for you. Since individually it is hard to tell which this is it will be something you may have to try for yourself before getting results.

Method 1: Leangains

This method is intended for those who spend a lot of time in the gym, it focuses on losing fat and building muscle and was created by Martain

Berkhan. If you aren't trying to gain muscle this might be a problem because many who want to lose weight do not want to become muscular.

The program advocates fasting for 14-16 hours a day though during this time you are allowed black coffee, sugar-free gum, calorie free soda and water. Essentially you are allowing yourself very tiny amounts of calories the FDA considers any product that has less than 5 calories a serving as being calorie free since your body needs to consume more than that to process the food. Most people find the easiest way to follow this is simply too fast through the night and morning, though they are still able to have their morning coffee as usual.

During the remaining 6-8 hours participants can "feed" and this will change depending on what days you exercise. On the days where you work out you will need to consume a higher level of carbs while on rest days you will need a higher level of fats. Your protein consumption should remain constant and high – the expected level is approximately

20g/day. If you aren't a nutritionist it is easy to see where an app like Calorie Counter might be essential until you get the hang of things. The foods you consume should also be whole and unprocessed as much as possible though this is a basic understanding of any healthy diet.

There are some pros and cons to this method. Firstly if you don't have time for a meal the program allows you to have a protein or nutritional shake instead though this is not intended to be a regular feature since it can push your body too far by having too few calories.

Another benefit is that there is no set meal time within the feeding schedule you may eat the entire 6-8 hour span within reason though many will still schedule 2-3 meals within that time.

Though so far you might think this is an easy program the emphasis with lean gains is what you eat. The guidelines within what you can eat are fairly strict and you will need to go over them in depth to make sure all your foods are within that parameter.

Time Windows

It is up to you to choose when your time window takes place, but it is recommended to time it smart and stay consistent with your time window. It is important to keep it sustainable, so you need to set the time window on moments that suit you well. For example, if you are someone who goes to the gym every morning, it will not be very smart to stuff yourself full right before you go.

Or if you are someone who has a 9-5 job, I wouldn't recommend taking in all your calories while you are working, as this can prevent you from staying focused on your work. Also, we are creatures of habit, so use this to your advantage.

Decide beforehand on which moment your time window will start each day, and stay consistent with that time window! Sticking to the program will be harder when you aren't consistent, due to the fact that you are repeatedly breaking the habit and because you aren't giving yourself the opportunity to form the habit in the first place.

Types of Food

What type of foods you eat depends on your goals, body fat, age and gender. Generally, you should eat a lot of protein, even on non-workout days. However, don't consume too much, as this could lead to protein toxicity. It is important to eat more carbohydrates than fats on training days, but lower your overall carbohydrate consumption when you are trying to lose body fat. Regardless of your goals, you should eat whole and unprocessed foods the majority of the time. You can occasionally have cheat days, but do this in moderation.

Benefits of Leangains

• Saves Money

When you are skipping certain meals for breakfast and lunch, this will provide a good opportunity to save money. Many people underestimate the amount of money they spend on breakfast and lunch every day.

• No Counting Calories

When you choose to eat in a short time window or eat all of your calories in one or two meals, it will become extremely hard to consume too many calories (if you are not eating junk food). Therefore, you will save yourself the trouble of micromanaging your calorie intake every time.

• Burns Fat

When you are following the Leangains diet, you will automatically eat less carbohydrates than normal. This will result in burning a lot of body fat. Your body will adapt to the fact that you aren't eating a lot of carbohydrates and it will burn the fat you have in order to receive energy.

Cons of Leangains

Leangains provides much flexibility when it comes to when you eat, but is very strict in the kind of foods you can eat. Most of the time this won't be a problem for active gym addicts, because the most committed are disciplined when it comes to nutrition.

Method 2: The Warrior Diet

This diet is ideal for those who like to outperform and dedicate to their goals. The language of the diet is very simple and the process even simpler. This is great for those who are very busy or who don't want to expend any time or effort adjusting their life to a diet. This diet has no feeding periods, or restrictions and is geared more towards those who feel comfortable undereating. In fact the problem with the Warrior Diet is that many people may find themselves in starvation as it is too extreme for those who aren't in the average range.

The program involves a 20 day fast and then a 4 hour period in which to eat a single large meal. However, during the 20 days fast you are allowed a few servings of raw veggies, fresh juice, and lean protein if desired. In this way this isn't a traditional fasting diet like the others because you aren't wholly fasting and can consume food during the fast period. The intention here is that the undereating promotes alertness by affecting the Sympathetic Nervous System.

The overeating period that follows this maximizes the recuperation from the fast without causing the body to go into starvation since you have consumed minimal calories to keep the metabolism going. The program advocates eating at night to make the body produce hormones and burn fat during the day as much as possible. According to Ori Hofmekler, who created the diet, the order in which you eat foods during your food groups is more important than anything during the four hour period. He advocates eating vegetables, followed by proteins, and then fats and only then if you are hungry resorting to carbohydrates.

This is by far one of the most popular fasting diets as it still allows participants to eat during the fasting period and isn't a true fast. Many have also said they really do feel more alert and have more energy by practicing this method. It seems this diet has a lot more pros than the others but yet again it falls short in that the eating period is quite strict, especially the order of eating. In addition it is also easy to overeat or at the very least consume far too many calories since you are eating during the day and then eating a bigger meal at night.

If your BMR is quite low this might be a disaster for you since you could eat enough calories grazing during the day that your "large" evening meal isn't necessary. The strict scheduling can also cause problems socially since you may not be able to eat with others or have to eat in a different order. It's also going to be difficult to follow if you don't like large meals or don't like to eat a lot at night.

Benefits of the Warrior Diet

• Eating Snacks in the Fasting Windows

One of the main benefits of this diet is that you can occasionally eat in your fasting window. You can consume fruits, veggies and fruit juice.

• Very Healthy

Another benefit of this diet is that you are getting all the nutrients you need on a daily basis. Cons of the Warrior Diet This diet can be very hard to sustain due to the fact that it is very strict on when and what to eat. Not many people can afford to eat at night, and some people find it very hard to consistently eat healthily.

Method 3: Eat and Stop

This method is quite difficult for those beginning fasting, especially if one of the reasons you have for being overweight is grazing. The stop phase of this program involves a 24 hour fast, and though at the beginning you are allowed to acclimatize to it eventually you are expected to go for the full 24 hours.

The idea behind this is that you are restricting your overall weekly calorie intake without having to limit what you're eating at all the rest of the time. This program also advocates resistance training as an exercise to maximize benefits. Similarly to the Leangains program you are still allowed calorie-free drinks like diet soda and coffee though no gum. There is no set schedule here so you can time your fast however you please – if you choose to finish your fast with a meal or a small snack is unimportant as long as you have completed the 24 hour period.

Though 24 hours may seem excessive the flexibility of this program can make this an easier program for beginners since you have no food restrictions. The creator, Brad Pilon, suggests spending the first day fasting for as long as you can before eating and then gradually extending that time each week until you reach your goal. He also suggests starting the fast at a time when you are busy so that you don't notice your lack of eating so much. Though there is no set dietary requirements it is still expected that you will eat healthy on your non-fasting days and the 24 hours is simply intended as and extra boost to lowering your calories on the other days.

The biggest con of this method is obviously the extended time without food. Most people will struggle with headaches, stomach cramps, fatigue, and becoming obnoxious simply because of hunger. In fact many people do get angry and cranky when hungry so it can be tempting to binge to get rid of this but this period is all about self-control. If you are nervous about how well you can control yourself over this period then this diet may be too challenging to follow. In other words this isn't meant for the casual dieter, this is more aimed towards those who already have a healthy lifestyle but need an extra boost to get to their weight loss goals.

Benefits of Eat Stop Eat

• Calorie Deficit Without Willpower Usage

Because you are limiting eating for just one or two days, it won't require any (or a lot of) willpower. When you know that you can eat what you want after enduring the 24-hour fast, it will be much easier to stick to it.

• Eat What You Want

You can also eat what you want, when you want, so this will help to prevent those nasty binges. The only thing is, moderation is key. You should only consume bad foods in moderation. Having one or two hands of chips is totally fine, but eating a bag of chips a day is not.

Cons of Eat Stop Eat

It can be hard to be disciplined in the Eat Stop Eat diet, even when you can eat what you want. Some people have a hard time eating bad food in moderation or binge on the days they can eat. If you find yourself struggling with a lack of self-control, then I wouldn't recommend this method to you.

Method 4: Up Day Down/The Alternate Day Diet

This is probably the easiest plan of the five here and is designed for those aiming to reach and maintain a specific goal. The program advocates eating very little one day followed by a normal intake the next day. If you are using the average 2000 calorie day as a guide this would mean your fast day should be between 400 to 500 calories. There is also a conveniently available tool online from the Dr. James Johnson who created the diet to calculate this based on your needs.

The doctor also advocates meal replacement products like shakes and bars on low-calorie days to maximize your nutritional intake on those. These products are also easier to ration out during the day than trying to calculate food amounts and needs then breaking them down to ration. The idea behind this is that once you have started to get the hang of rationing yourself, you can begin to transition over to regular foods on your fast days while still keeping in the guided amount.

As a method this is the most well supported,probably because it has been formulated by a doctor. This program gives you the necessary ~30% calorie reduction while giving you about a 1-2% weight loss per week (around 2lb for most people). However it can be easy to "forget" you're dieting on those alternate days which could cause binging and the diet to fail. The plan does advocate meal planning as well so that you don't find yourself in this situation or being forced into fast food.

One of the most notable differences with this diet is that it does not advocate fast results but a more sustained rate over time, this can be frustrating and many will feel they are not getting results or that the diet isn't working.

Each of these methods has pros and cons, and with any weight loss method you may not see immediate results which is why it is important to stick with it. If you struggle with the timing of the meals or cannot stretch yourself to fast for as long as the diets require you can also consider programs like the Primal Diet or Intuitive eating. Eat WHEN for example trains dieters to listen to when their body gives them cues about when to eat. If you're a grazer by nature though this is an easy path to overeating and it may simply be time to master your willpower and work with an intermittent fasting method.

Benefits of this method

• Rapid Weight Loss

Due the fact that you are cutting a lot of calories every day, you will see results very fast. Many people report that they lose about 1-2 pounds a week.

• Eat What You Prefer

There is no restriction on what to eat, but it is advised to eat unprocessed and whole foods. However, you may only eat the maximum amount of calories you need to maintain your weight on the normal calorie days.

• Doesn't Require Much Willpower

Because you are only cutting calories for 2-3 days a week, you won't use too much willpower. It can be difficult at first, but it is better to start the diet very small. Start by cutting a few calories out on the low-calorie days and gradually keep increasing this.

Method 5: Fast/Feast method

If you're a fan of cheat days this could be the one for you, the other diets have advocated snacking or drinks as cheats during your fasting period while this one actually combines all three and then still allows you one cheat day a week. The rest of the week is then split up using different methods of fasting. As with the EatStopEat program the creators suggest using your busiest time as your fasting period so you don't realize you're fasting as much.

Unlike the other plans, however this one also has a companion training program for participants to maximize the results they have as easily as possible. In this way even though you aren't following as strict of a dietary regime it is a higher impact on your lifestyle since you will need to follow an exercise regime too. The biggest bonus of using this method is that for those who aren't good at planning out or scheduling eating times this program has everything already scheduled out for you. Conveniently this allows you to have your cheat day while still giving you structure and maximum rewards.

The opposite of this is that one cheat day can often turn into two and then the whole program fails so though it doesn't require as much willpower as EatStopEat it does mean that you will need enough to keep your cheating in check. Also since the planned schedule varies on a daily basis there is not a lot of room for flexibility and it can be inconvenient to fit into a busy lifestyle. The calendar provided with the program will provide some help but it is still the largest impact on your day compared to the other programs.

Benefits of this method

• Fat Loss

By fasting for 36 hours, you are taking in a lower amount of calories. This will lead to a rapid fat loss.

• Full Cheat Days

The Fast/Feast Model allows you to implement full cheat days. This is excellent for the common sweet tooth and it helps you to keep your metabolism working.

• Removes Food Cravings

By implementing cheat days, it becomes easier to resist unhealthy foods along the way. It will give your body a mental and physical break. Removing food cravings will help you to avoid overeating junk food.

Cons of this method

The method is relatively difficult to follow due to the following two reasons:

• Very Difficult To Keep Your Calories In Check

For most people it will become very difficult to keep their calories in check during their cheat days.

If you are unfamiliar with the amount of calories that most foods contain, it is almost impossible to not cross your limit too much.

• 36-Hour Fasts Can Be Very Long

If you have never fasted before, it can be very difficult to sustain the 36-hour fast. Most people who do this version of Intermittent Fasting are already familiar and advanced with it, which is why they are able to sustain it easier.

However, like the Alternate Day Diet, start this model by beginning small. Don't try to fast for 36 hours at once, but rather begin small by fasting for 12 hours and gradually increase the time.

Chapter 10: Efficiency in Intermittent Fasting

I remember that when I started, I made some critical mistakes which slowed down the process of implementing Intermittent Fasting. I want to show you exactly how to implement Intermittent Fasting efficiently without making unnecessary mistakes.

Step #1: Start With The Why

With everything you do in life, you should know the reasons behind it. Doing certain things without knowing exactly why you are doing them will eventually cause you to fail. The same goes with Intermittent Fasting. Before you even start to implement it, you need to know why you want to implement Intermittent Fasting. Our Different Personalities Ok, how do you do this? We human beings have different personalities (or different selves). We have a lower, a standard and a higher self. We tend to switch between these personalities throughout the day, depending on the time, place, situation and environment we are in.

Every one of these personalities is motivated by different things and you need to align all these personalities to the same goal: implementing Intermittent Fasting. And when your goal (to implement Intermittent Fasting) is not aligned between these personalities, you will eventually sabotage yourself. Therefore, the key is to come up with reasons that are emotionally compelling to you for all your personalities to achieve a particular goal.

For example, let's say that you are in a standard mood; you suddenly decide to lose 10 pounds of body fat and your motivation is because you want to look good. You realize that you need to change your eating patterns, so you go on a diet. Well, it is very good to go on a diet, and "looking good" is a very good reason to lose body fat.

However, there is one problem… you only know why your standard self-wants to lose 10 pounds of body fat. But what about your higher self or your lower self? Why do 'they' want to lose the body fat? What if you catch yourself in a stressed-out mood and crave some junk food? You will most likely think "screw this diet" and sabotage yourself. Or when you are in a higher self, you don't specifically care about looking good, so you think "why to bother?"

How To Recognize Our Different Personalities

So again, the key is to come up with reasons that are emotionally compelling to you for all your personalities. And how do you recognize your different selves? Simple, by the thought patterns you have. Normally, when you have negative thought patterns, you tend to be in your lower self. When you have neutral thoughts, you are in your standard self, and if you have very positive thoughts, you are in your higher self. Your Lower Self: Tends to be motivated by selfish, irrational and slightly more childish reasons being better than others, showing people a lesson, being lazy, avoiding responsibility etc.

Your Standard Self: Tends to be motivated by logical, rational and ethical reasons like: knowing that you need to do XYZ to get a certain result, realizing your responsibility etc.

Your Higher Self: Tends to be motivated by a sense of higher purpose like: motivating and inspiring others, having a positive impact on the world, contributing to society etc.

Exercise: Determine Your Own Reasons To Implement Intermittent Fasting

Now that you know how to create your own reasons for implementing Intermittent Fasting, it is time for you to determine them. Take 10 minutes to a half hour to sit down and come up with all the reasons why you want/ need to implement Intermittent

Fasting. I have showed you all the benefits of Intermittent Fasting and I also showed you that the most common myths about Intermittent Fasting simply aren't true. Now, take the time to look at the reasons which compel you the most.

Also, come up with other personal reasons to implement Intermittent Fasting. These reasons need to be emotionally compelling to you and move you towards your goal. Also, only having negative or positive reasons for implementing Intermittent Fasting is not good enough. You need to have both (and even logical reasons).

Again, take 10 minutes to a half hour to come up with reasons for your lower self, standard self and higher self. Be sure to come up with as many reasons as possible!

Step #2: Choose Which Intermittent Fasting Model You

Want To Implement, we have discussed several Intermittent Fasting Models that you can implement. These models are very similar, but differ in the actual execution. Again, which model you should implement is completely up to you, but it depends on your goals. You need to clearly define your goals and check which Intermittent Fasting model is the best choice for your personal goal.

You can, of course, also mix the concepts of these Intermittent Fasting models. For example, I have implemented a variation of the Leangains model and the Alternate Day Diet model. I really like the concept of the Leangains model, but there are some things that aren't practical for me. So, I decided to create little modifications to the model by mixing it with the Alternate Day Diet model. To be honest though, I don't recommend you create a variation of the models if you are new to Intermittent Fasting.

I recommend that you first choose a model, execute it and see what happens. If you find that it isn't practical for you, then it may be smart to make some small tweaks to the model or try to implement another one.

Step #3: Divide The Principles Of Your Chosen Model Into Habits You Can Implement

These habits are discussed in the next chapter, Chapter 11. Again, everything we human beings do in life is a learned habit. Habits can be our greatest asset or our greatest liability. For example, someone who is exercising daily has formed a great habit (read: asset). But someone who is eating junk food every day has formed a very disturbing habit (read: liability). You want to form great habits that will help you to move forward towards your goals.

But implementing these habits can be very difficult, because it demands willpower to create a habit. So what you'll want to do is to divide all the principles into tiny habits that you can implement easily. At first it will feel as if you aren't making any progress, but I can assure you that you will if you do it consistently.

Also, don't make the mistake of trying to implement too many habits at once. You have a limited amount of willpower and when you implement too many habits, you will burn through all your willpower very fast, resulting in you sabotaging your progress or discarding the whole Intermittent Fasting model.

Step #4: Review And Visualize Your Habits plus Implement One A Month

To properly implement the habits chosen in step 3, you need to implement them very slowly. I know a lot of people want to make change very quick, so they decide to overhaul their diet within a week. This is not the correct way to do it! No matter how much willpower you have, every human being has a breaking point. The breaking point is the point where you burn out all your willpower and discard all your chosen habits. When that happens, you are not making progress, or worse, you are actually going backward!

Chapter 11: Habits that can be adapted for Successful fasting

To make it easier to you, I have divided all the Intermittent Fasting models from chapter 3 into tiny habits here below:

Leangains

Habit 1: Starting your eating window on X hour (the moment you want to start your eating window daily).

Habit 2: Break your eating window on X+8 hours (8 hours after you have started your eating window).

Habit 3A (For people trying to lose weight): Eat 25% carbohydrates, 40% protein, and 35% fat of your total daily calorie consumption.

Habit 3B (For people trying to gain weight): Eat 50% carbohydrates, 35% protein, and 15% fat of your total daily calorie consumption. Make sure you eat approximately 200-400 more calories than shown to properly gain weight.

The Warrior Diet

Habit 1: Starting your eating window on X hour (the moment you want to start your eating window daily, but it has to be in the night).

Habit 2: Break your eating window on X+4 hours (4 hours after you have started your eating window).

Habit 3: Replace bad snacks (processed foods etc.) with fruits

Habit 4: Start eating small portions of the protein outside your eating window (around 100 calories per meal).

Habit 5: Replace bad drinks (soft drinks etc.) with fruit juice and water.

Eat Stop Eat

Habit 1: Choose a day where you want to fast for 24 hours and start by fasting for 12 hours on that day.

Habit 2: Increase your fast to 16 hours on that day.

Habit 3: Increase your fast to 20 hours on that day.

Habit 4: Increase your fast to 24 hours on that day.

Habit 5 (for people who want to fast for 24 hours on another day): Repeat habit #1 to habit #4 for another day.

Alternate Day Diet

First, determine how many calories you need to sustain your weight.

Habit 1: Make sure that you consume the amount of calories needed to sustain your weight every day.

Habit 2: Eat 80% of your calories on low-calorie days.

Habit 3: Decrease that to 60% of your calories on low-calorie days.

Habit 4: Decrease that to 40% of your calories on low-calorie days.

Habit 5: Decrease that to 20% of your calories on low-calorie days.

Fast/Feast Model

Habit 1: Endure a 12-hour fast followed by a normal day of eating

Habit 2: Endure an 18-hour fast followed by a normal day of eating

Habit 3: Endure a 24-hour fast followed by a normal day of eating

Habit 4: Endure a 32-hour fast followed by a cheat day

Habit 5: Endure a 36-hour fast followed by a cheat day How to Implement A Habit

So how do you implement habits without burning out all your willpower?

Implement one habit a month. For example, decide that you are going to execute habit 1 on day 1 all the way to day 30. If you have done that successfully, you may proceed to implement habit 2. If you catch yourself failing to execute habit 1 somewhere between day 1 and day 30, restart the cycle. I know that it sounds very boring and annoying to do, but this is the only way to do it effectively.

Also, realize that the more you do something, the easier it gets. Only the first week or two will be the toughest, and after that you can be almost 100% sure that you will follow through.

Another thing to consider is that if you have implemented the first habit successfully, but you catch yourself failing to execute it while trying to implement habit 2, you need to go back and start the 30 days over with habit 1.

The goal is not to do every habit for 30 days once, but rather to sustain those habits. Therefore, always make sure that the habits you implemented earlier are being carried out while doing the newer ones.

Review and Visualize Your Habits.

Also, you need to take approximately 10 minutes a day to effectively review and visualize yourself doing the habits. If you do this, you will constantly remind yourself why you are doing what you are doing and help yourself to make the habit a part of your reality.

To effectively review your habit, read the reasons why you want to implement those habits.

After that, take 7-10 minutes to visualize doing the habit successfully.

Chapter 12: What can cause failure in Intermittent Fasting

Many people may fail to sustain fasting. In this chapter, we are going to look at some of the factors that may cause individuals to be unsuccessful in making a good and required fast.

Reason #1: Your Reasons Aren't Strong Enough

As stated earlier, you need to come up with several compelling reasons to implement Intermittent Fasting into your life. If you don't have enough reasons that emotionally compel you at all times, you will be more likely to fail. Also, there is a chance that people will question your decision and if you aren't able to fully explain to yourself exactly why you need to implement Intermittent Fasting, at some point you will think: "Why bother? Screw this."

Solution:

The solution is very simple - state at least 15 reasons that emotionally compel you on why you should Intermittent Fast. This will help you to stick to it, even when people question your behavior.

Reason #2: Going Too Hard

Even if you are doing everything right, the chances are that you are still failing to sustain your Intermittent Fasting diet. Why? Because you are trying to implement all the habits at once. While I understand that you want to implement Intermittent Fasting into your life quickly, it isn't the smartest way to go about it. We as human beings have a limited amount of willpower, and every time you try to implement a new habit, you use up a bit.

So, you can understand that if you try to implement them all at once, you will deplete all of your willpower very quickly. When this happens, you have reached your breaking point. When you have reached your breaking point, you will most likely give up on Intermittent Fasting and go back in doing things the old way. Or worse, you there will be a chance that you will develop bad habits.

Solution:

As discussed earlier, you need to identify whether you are a slow learner or a fast learner. How fast are you able to implement things? This is a question you can only answer by experimenting with it. Begin small and gradually, then increase a number of habits you take on.

Realize that everyone has a breaking point and everyone will give up when they have reached this breaking point. If you catch yourself giving up eventually, even while doing everything right, choose to apply the habits a bit slower than you had planned to. See the implementation of Intermittent Fasting as a marathon, not a sprint.

Slow but steady will always win the race. It is the person who implements things slowly but consistently who succeeds, as opposed to the person who goes all out for the first 2 weeks and quits after that. In short, take it one step at a time and stay consistent.

Reason #3 Too Many Distractions

To quote Jim Rohn, "You are the average of the 5 people you spend the most time with." With this quote, Jim Rohn is trying to say that you will take on the habits of the people you spend the most time with, whether you like it or not. This is because we human beings are social creatures and one of our primal desires is to belong to a group of people.

But also (as discussed earlier), you just have as much willpower that you can use to sustain your own habits when you are with these 5 people. If you are someone who eats healthy all the time, but your 5 people are junk food addicts, it won't take too long until you catch yourself eating junk food regularly.

These 5 people can be a blessing or a curse to your goals. If they have the same goals as you, it will become a lot easier to succeed. If this is not the case, you will set yourself up for failure. Therefore, there might be a chance that you aren't able to stick with Intermittent Fasting due to these people.

Solutio:

The first thing you need to realize is that it isn't their fault that you aren't succeeding with Intermittent Fasting. It is just that your and their goals are in conflict. A way to get around this is by asking them if they want to help you with the issue. Explain to them why Intermittent Fasting is so important to you and show them what results it brings you. Ask them if they can respect your decision and whether they can eat at different moments if you are around.

I personally asked my friends to bear in mind that it was very difficult for me to stick to fasting when they would consistently eat around me, and I rarely had any issues with them. Even the individual who stated that it was a waste of my time was still able to respect me by eating elsewhere when I was around. If some people really don't want to cooperate, choose to remove yourself from their presence when they eat. In short, eliminate all distractions. As stated earlier, you need to come up with several compelling reasons to implement Intermittent Fasting into your life. If you don't have enough reasons that emotionally compel you at all times, you will be more likely to fail.

Conclusion

Congratulations, you've reached the end of Intermittent Fasting! I hope you know a lot more about fasting and that you (if you haven't already) will start implementing Intermittent Fasting into your life. Now that you know that fasting provides a lot of benefits, is easy to implement and that the common myths aren't true, I hope you are motivated to implement the information.

The truth is with intermittent fasting there really isn't one as it is much easier to do than it first seems. To lose weight with intermittent fasting you don't change your healthy eating habits at all except for one or two 24 hour periods each week where you don't consume any calories. These facts should be scheduled to make them as easy as possible. When not fasting you just eat what you normally would. Ideally this should feature good quality meats and fish with mostly fibrous, not starchy or sweet carbohydrates plus a lot of drinking water. Just don't eat waste your fast be eating extra to make up for it! Don't fast more than twice per week or for longer than 24 hours at any one time.

The intermittent fasting program can be very effective, safe and sustainable. One of the best benefits of IF is that once you have the program in place you can carry it on for life. You do not need special food or to buy special supplements or a special program, you can eat what you normally eat just at a scheduled timeframe.

Unlike a fad diet, which only works for a short period of time, the intermittent fasting method can be a lifestyle. You can eat real food and get all the nutrients you need. There are no restrictions. A key to remember with any program is that there are no true shortcuts, all the programs at the beginning will be difficult because they are forcing you to change. But with the intermittent fasting method if you stick to it and make it your lifestyle you will not have the problem of the yo-yo effect (going up and down in weight).

One thing that I recommend is that you should always consult with a physician or nutritionist before starting this or any program that involves changes in your nutrition or involves a change in your exercise regimen.

Thank you for taking the time to join me in this in this journey of understanding intermittent fasting. Fasting can make people achieve a lot in life. So know the essence of taking a fast and good luck in all your fasting endeavors.